Biochemistry Research Trends

Analytical Chemistry and Microchemistry

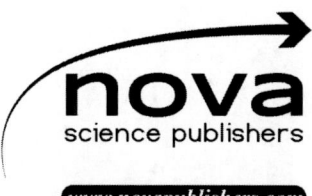

Biochemistry Research Trends

The Medical Biology Guide to Proteins
David Aebisher, PhD, DSc (Editor)
2023. ISBN: 979-8-88697-910-7 (Softcover)
2023. ISBN: 979-8-89113-024-1 (eBook)

Water in Biology: A Molecular View
Michael E. Green, PhD (Editor)
Alisher M Kariev (Editor)
2023. ISBN: 979-8-88697-708-0 (Hardcover)
2023. ISBN: 979-8-88697-754-7 (eBook)

More information about this series can be found at
https://novapublishers.com/product-category/series/biochemistry-research-trends/

Analytical Chemistry and Microchemistry

Modern Approaches in Fluid Chromatography: Impact and Applications
Rohit Bhatia, PhD and Bhupinder Kumar, PhD (Editors)
2023. ISBN: 979-8-88697-856-8 (Hardcover)
2023. ISBN: 979-8-89113-022-7 (eBook)

Chromatographic Methods and Research
Raven W. Obrien (Editor)
2023. ISBN: 979-8-89113-193-4 (Hardcover)
2023. ISBN: 979-8-89113-203-0 (eBook)

More information about this series can be found at
https://novapublishers.com/product-category/series/analytical-chemistry-and-microchemistry/

Jimmy Hu, PhD

Airborne and Biological Monitoring to Assess Occupational Exposure to Isocyanates

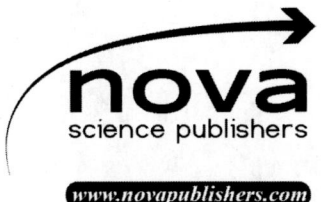

Copyright © 2023 by Nova Science Publishers, Inc.
https://doi.org/10.52305/NPTC8511

All rights reserved. No part of this book may be reproduced, stored in a retrieval system or transmitted in any form or by any means: electronic, electrostatic, magnetic, tape, mechanical photocopying, recording or otherwise without the written permission of the Publisher.

We have partnered with Copyright Clearance Center to make it easy for you to obtain permissions to reuse content from this publication. Please visit copyright.com and search by Title, ISBN, or ISSN.

For further questions about using the service on copyright.com, please contact:

	Copyright Clearance Center	
Phone: +1-(978) 750-8400	Fax: +1-(978) 750-4470	E-mail: info@copyright.com

NOTICE TO THE READER

The Publisher has taken reasonable care in the preparation of this book but makes no expressed or implied warranty of any kind and assumes no responsibility for any errors or omissions. No liability is assumed for incidental or consequential damages in connection with or arising out of information contained in this book. The Publisher shall not be liable for any special, consequential, or exemplary damages resulting, in whole or in part, from the readers' use of, or reliance upon, this material. Any parts of this book based on government reports are so indicated and copyright is claimed for those parts to the extent applicable to compilations of such works.

Independent verification should be sought for any data, advice or recommendations contained in this book. In addition, no responsibility is assumed by the Publisher for any injury and/or damage to persons or property arising from any methods, products, instructions, ideas or otherwise contained in this publication.

This publication is designed to provide accurate and authoritative information with regards to the subject matter covered herein. It is sold with the clear understanding that the Publisher is not engaged in rendering legal or any other professional services. If legal or any other expert assistance is required, the services of a competent person should be sought. FROM A DECLARATION OF PARTICIPANTS JOINTLY ADOPTED BY A COMMITTEE OF THE AMERICAN BAR ASSOCIATION AND A COMMITTEE OF PUBLISHERS.

Library of Congress Cataloging-in-Publication Data
Names: Hu, Jimmy, author.
Title: Airborne and biological monitoring to assess occupational exposure
    to isocyanates / Jimmy Hu, PhD.
Identifiers: LCCN 2023033268 (print) | LCCN 2023033269 (ebook) | ISBN
    9798891130104 (paperback) | ISBN 9798891130999 (adobe pdf)
Subjects: LCSH: Isocyanates--Safety measures. | Isocyanates--Threshold limit values. | Isocyanates--Toxicology. | Isocyanates--Industrial applications.
Classification: LCC TP248.I8 H85 2023 (print) | LCC TP248.I8 (ebook) |
    DDC 661/.8940289--dc23/eng/20230824
LC record available at https://lccn.loc.gov/2023033268
LC ebook record available at https://lccn.loc.gov/2023033269

Published by Nova Science Publishers, Inc. † New York

Contents

List of Figures ix

Preface xi

Acknowledgments xiii

Abbreviations xv

Chapter 1   **Isocyanates** 1
                1.1. Common Isocyanate Compounds   1
                1.2. Production and Reactivity   5
                1.3. Common Applications   6
                      1.3.1. Manufacturing of Isocyanates   7
                      1.3.2. Use in Manufacturing of PUs and PU Composite Materials   7
                      1.3.3. Use in Manufacture of Foams   8
                      1.3.4. Use in Spray Foam Applications   8
                      1.3.5. Use in Coatings   9
                      1.3.6. Use in Adhesives   9

Chapter 2   **Health and Safety** 11
                2.1. Introduction   11
                2.2. Hazard Statements   12
                2.3. Exposure Routes   13
                2.4. Risk Management   14
                      2.4.1. Exposure Controls   *14*
                      2.4.2. Exposure Standards   *19*
                      2.4.3. Regulation   *22*
                      2.4.4. Exposure Monitoring   *23*
                      2.4.5. Health Surveillance   *24*
                2.5. Conclusion   26

Chapter 3	Laboratory Analytical Methods	29
	3.1. Introduction	29
	3.2. Sample Preparation	31
	3.3. Analytical Techniques	32
	3.3.1. Gas Chromatography	*32*
	3.3.2. Flame Ionisation Detection	*33*
	3.3.3. Mass Spectrometer	*33*
	3.3.4. High-Performance Liquid Chromatography	*34*
	3.3.5. Ultra-Violet/Electrochemical Detections	*35*
	3.3.6. Tandem Mass Spectrometer	*36*
	3.4. Examples of Analytical Methods	40
	3.4.1. Method for Assessing Airborne Isocyanates as -NCO Group by LC-UV-ECD	*40*
	3.4.2. Method for Assessing Airborne Both Isocyanate Monomers and Oligomers by LC-MS-MS	*42*
	3.4.3. Method for Assessing Biomarkers of Exposure to Isocyanates by LC-MS/MS	*46*
	3.5. Laboratory Accreditation and Quality Control/Assurance	48
	3.6. Discussion	49
	3.6.1. Ultra/Violet and Electrochemical Detections Verse Mass Spectrometer	*49*
	3.6.2. Gas Chromatograph-Mass Spectrometer verse Liquid Chromatograph-Mass Spectrometer	*51*
	3.7. Conclusion	54
Chapter 4	Airborne Monitoring and Its Applications	57
	4.1. Introduction	57
	4.2. Sampling and Analytical Methods	59
	4.2.1. OSHA and NIOSH Methods	*59*
	4.2.2. Other Widely Used Methods	*61*
	4.3. Critical Areas to Focus on Improvement of Methods	64
	4.3.1. Sampling of Isocyanates (Impinger vs Filters)	*65*
	4.3.2. Derivatisation	*66*

Contents vii

	4.3.3. Monomers and oligomers	68
	4.3.4. Detection	69
	4.3.5. Continuous Monitoring Exposure Isocyanates Techniques	70
	4.4. Occupational Exposure to Isocyanates	72
	4.4.1. Manufacturing of Isocyanates	73
	4.4.2. Applications in the Manufacture of PUs and PU Composite Materials	74
	4.4.3. Applications in the Manufacture of Foams	75
	4.4.4. Applications in Spray Foam	76
	4.4.5. Applications in Coatings	77
	4.4.6. Applications in Adhesives	78
	4.4.7. Discussions	78
	4.5. Conclusion and Future Research Goals	80
Chapter 5	**Biological Monitoring and Its Applications**	81
	5.1. Introduction	81
	5.2. International Approaches	83
	5.3. Assessing Exposure (Regulation)	86
	5.4. Advantages and Disadvantages of Biological Monitoring	87
	5.5. Practical Approaches	89
	5.5.1. Common Media	89
	5.5.2. Sampling	90
	5.5.3. Analytical Methods	91
	5.5.4. Interpretation	98
	5.5.5. Criteria for Selection of a Biomarker	99
	5.6. Applications	104
	5.6.1. Monitoring Exposure to HDI	104
	5.6.2. Monitoring Exposure to TDI	109
	5.6.3. Monitoring Exposure to MDI	110
	5.7. Conclusion	115
References		119
Index		135
About the Author		141

List of Figures

Figure 1.1.	Chemical structures of selected isocyanates of major commercial values. (a) Aliphatic isocyanates and (b) Aromatic isocyanates	4
Figure 2.1.	A diagram of hierarchy of controls	15
Figure 2.2.	A simplified flow chart of health surveillance for the spray painters using paints containing isocyanates	25
Figure 3.1.	Relation of the molecular mass range and the polarity of analytes analysable by GC-MS and LC-MS interface techniques (APCI and ESI)	30
Figure 3.2.	Schematic diagram of Gas chromatograph-Mass Spectrometry	33
Figure 3.3.	Comparison of single quadrupole mass spectrometer (LC-MS) and triple quadrupole mass spectrometer (LC-MS/MS)	38
Figure 3.4.	The chromatogram of LC-UV (A) LC-ECD and (B) of 2,6-TDI and MDI 1,2-MP derivatives	41
Figure 3.5.	The application of LC-MS/MS is used in the analysis of isocyanates by air monitoring	44
Figure 3.6.	LC-MS/MS chromatograms of work-up urine samples spiked with amines at 10 µg/L and with the deuterium-labelled amines at 5 µg/L	45
Figure 4.1.	Common sampling methods for isocyanates.	58
Figure 4.2.	CIP 10 (CDL, carrefour du laboratorie) air sampler and the polyurethane foam creates the air flow and collects the dust	70

List of Figures

Figure 5.1. The link between external exposure, internal dose and biological response and their relationship with different types of occupational limit values (BEL, OEL, BLV). Modified from the "Guidelines on Biological Monitoring" of the Italian Society of Occupational Medicine and Industrial Hygiene 86

Figure 5.2. Interpretation of biological monitoring results 98

Figure 5.3. Molecular structure of HDA Isocyanuarate as a biomarker for HDI Isocyanuarate 101

Figure 5.4. Molecular structure of acetyl-MDI-Lysine as a biomarker for MDI 102

Figure 5.5. Molecular structure of HDI-Lysine as a biomarker for HDI 103

Preface

This book serves as an essential guide for professionals working in industries that use isocyanates - a widely used compound in the manufacturing of polyurethanes, foams, coatings, adhesives, and other materials. The book provides a comprehensive understanding of airborne and biological monitoring techniques for reducing occupational exposure to isocyanates. The intended audience includes occupational hygienists and analytical chemists with basic knowledge of occupational hygiene and chemistry.

Starting with a comprehensive overview of common isocyanate compounds, their production, reactivity, and applications, the book highlights the potential health hazards posed to workers. Chapter 2 delves into the importance of health and safety measures to protect workers from isocyanate exposure. It provides an in-depth analysis of exposure routes, risk management, exposure controls, exposure standards, and regulatory requirements. The chapter also offers practical insights into achieving adequate control, exposure monitoring, and health surveillance.

Chapter 3 offers a detailed description of laboratory analytical methods, including sample preparation, analytical techniques, laboratory accreditation, quality control/assurance, and different detection methods. Chapter 4 focuses on workplace air sampling, analysis, and applications, highlighting critical areas for improvement such as sampling, derivatization, detection, and continuous monitoring exposure techniques. It also covers occupational exposure to isocyanates in various manufacturing applications.

Chapter 5 focuses on biological sampling, analytical methods, and applications for assessing exposure to isocyanates. It discusses international approaches, assessing exposure regulation, advantages and disadvantages of biological monitoring, practical approaches, common biological media, sampling, analytical methods, interpretation, criteria for selection of a biomarker, and future perspectives.

The book is a valuable resource for professionals in the manufacturing industry, occupational health and safety professionals, researchers, laboratory chemists, and students. It provides a detailed and practical understanding of the potential health hazards of isocyanates, how to assess exposure, and how to implement effective exposure controls and monitoring techniques to ensure worker safety.

Acknowledgments

I would like to express my heartfelt gratitude to several individuals and organizations for their invaluable contributions to this book.

First and foremost, I want to acknowledge the efforts of Mr Robbie Geyer, my lab manager, and Dr. Greg O'Donnell, my QA manager at SafeWork NSW, for their instrumental role in developing the method for biological monitoring of isocyanate exposure in the workplace. I am also grateful for their ongoing support throughout this project.

Furthermore, I would like to recognize Dr. John Cocker and Ms. Kate Jones from the Health and Safety Laboratory in the UK, for inspiring the development of the commercial method for biological monitoring of isocyanate exposure in Australia during their visit to my laboratory at SafeWork NSW. I also extend my appreciation to Ms. Ana Milosavljevic and Ms. Sally North from WorkSafe WA for their cooperation during the preliminary field testing of the method.

My special thanks go to Mr. Aklesh Nand, Manager of Hygiene & Toxicology Chemicals, Explosives, and Safety Auditing, and Dr. Phillip Cantrell, State Inspector, both from SafeWork NSW, for their successful application of the developed analytical method to assess isocyanate exposure in the motor vehicle repair industry in NSW, Australia.

I am also grateful to Ms. Lisa Hunt, the CEO of WorkCover NSW, for awarding the Chairman's Award to the project of biological monitoring to assess exposure to isocyanates. I also extend my appreciation to the AIOH for awarding the presentation as 3M Best Conference Paper at the 2010 AIOH Conference in Hobart, Australia. These internal and external awards provided the encouragement and motivation to continue developing the project to a world-class level that has been recognized internationally.

Finally, I would like to express my love and gratitude to my family, Linda, Tina, and Serena, for their unwavering support and encouragement throughout this endeavour.

Abbreviations

ACGIH	American Conference of Governmental Industrial Hygienists
AIHA	American Industrial Hygiene Association
AIOH	Australian Institute of Occupational Hygienists
APCI	Atmospheric Pressure Chemical Ionization
ASTM	American Society for Testing and Materials
BAT	Biologische Arbeitsstoff Toleranzwerte (biological tolerance values)
BEI	Biological Exposure Index
BMGV	Biological Monitoring Guidance Value
BGV	Biological Guidance Value
COH	Certified Occupational Hygienist
CSRs	Chemical Safety Reports
DAD	Diode Array Detector
DAN	1,8-Diaminonaphtalene
DBA	Dibutylamine
DFG	Deutsche Forschungsgemeinschaft
ECD	Electrochemical Detection
ECHA	European Chemicals Agency
EPA	Environmental Protection Agency, USA
ESI	Electrospray Ionisation
EU	European Union
FID	Flame Ionisation Detection
FLD	Fluorescence detection
GC	Gas Chromatography
G-EQUAS	German External QUality Assessment Scheme
HCIS	Hazardous Chemical Information System
HCOTN	Health Council of the Netherlands
HDA	Hexamethylene Diamine
HDI	Hexamethylene Diisocyanate

HPLC	High-Performance Liquid Chromatography
HSE	Health & Safety Executive, UK
HSL	Health & Safety Laboratory, UK
IARC	International Agency for Research on Cancer
IEC	The International Electrotechnical Commission
IPDI	Isophorone Diisocyanate
ISO	International Standards Organization
LC	Liquid Chromatography
LC-MS	Liquid Chromatography–Mass Spectrometry
LC-MS/MS	Liquid Chromatography with Tandem Mass Spectrometry
LLE	Liquid-Liquid Extraction
L/min	Litres per minute
LOD	Limit of Detection
LOQ	Limit of Quantitation
MAMA	(N-methyl-aminomethyl)anthracene
MAP	1-(9-anthracenylmethyl)piperazine
MDA	Methylene Diphenyl Diamine
MDHS	Methods for the Determination of Hazardous Substance, HSE, UK
MDI	Methylene Diphenyl Isocyanate
mg/m^3	milligrams (10^{-3} grams) per cubic metre
MOPIP	1-(2-methoxyphenyl)-piperazine
1,2-MP	1-(2-methoxyphenyl)-piperazine
MRM	Multiple Reaction Monitoring
MS	Mass Spectrometer
MVR	Motor Vehicle Repair
NATA	National Association of Testing Authorities, Australia
NCO	Isocyanate functional group; Nitrogen=Carbon=Oxygen
NIOSH	National Institute for Occupational Safety and Health, USA
NIST	The National Institute of Standards and Technology, USA
Nitro reagent	p-nitrobenzyl-N-propylamine
NMR	Nuclear Magnetic Resonance
NOHSC	National Occupational Safety and Health Commission, Australia
OEL	Occupational Exposure Limit
OSHA	Occupational Safety & Health Agency, USA
PAT	Proficiency Analytical Testing
PDA	Photodiode Array Detector
PELs	Permissible Exposure Limits

1,2-PP	1-(2-pyridyl)-piperazine
PPE	Personal Protective Equipment
ppm	parts per million
PT	Proficiency Test
PTFE	Polytetrafluoroethylene
PU	Polyurethane
QC/QA	Quality Control/Quality Assurance
SCOEL	Scientific Committee on Occupational Exposure Limits
SDS	Safety Data Sheet
SPE	Solid Phase Extraction
STEL	Short-term Exposure Limit
SWA	Safe Work Australia
TDA	Toluene Diamine
TDI	Toluene Diisocyanate
TEA	Time Weighted Average
TLV	Threshold Limit Value
TOF	Time-of-Flight
TRIG	Total Reactive Isocyanate Group
UK	United Kingdom
UPLC	Ultra-Performance Liquid Chromatography
US	United States of America
UV	Ultra-violet
$\mu g/m^3$	micrograms (10^{-6} grams) per cubic metre
WES	Workplace Exposure Standard

Chapter 1

Isocyanates

1.1. Common Isocyanate Compounds

Isocyanate is the functional group with the formula R-N=C=O. Organic compounds that contain an isocyanate group are referred to as isocyanates. The NCO unit that defines isocyanates is planar, and the NCO linkage is nearly linear.

Isocyanates are categorized depending on the number of isocyanate functional groups, such as monoisocyanate, diisocyanate, triisocyanate and polyisocyanate. Diisocyanates are the smallest base unit that can allow polymerization. Oligomers (also called polyisocyanates) are small polymers composed from only a small number of monomeric units, whereas prepolymers are generally composed of larger polymer chains containing two or more isocyanate groups. The commercial products used in numerous processes are generally made up of diisocyanates and oligomers. Note that in this book, the term "isocyanate" will be used to designate any compound having at least two isocyanate groups. The abbreviation, full name, CAS number, molecular weight, and chemical structure of widely used isocyanates are listed and demonstrated in Figure 1.1.

Like common chemicals, the vapour pressure of isocyanates decreases with increasing molecular weight. HDI and TDI have low vapour pressures of 0.01 and 0.02 mm Hg at 20°C, respectively, while MDI, HMDI, polymeric MDI and polymeric HDI have very low vapour pressures of less than 0.0000075 mm Hg at 20°C. Manufacturer's products are therefore designed to include high percentages of oligomer and pre-polymer compounds to achieve the lowest vapour pressure possible. Spray painting formulations have a high proportion of polymeric HDI (usually > 60%) with the monomer component being usually less than 1% [Dulux, 2021a; Dulux, 2021b]. Foam formulations using MDI usually have a monomer content of about 40 to 50%, with the remainder being made up of an equal amount of polymeric MDI oligomer [IARC 1999]. Therefore, isocyanates are not very volatile at room temperature. However, increased temperature will result in an increase in vapour pressure and a rise in the concentration of these chemicals in the vapour phase. Spraying promotes the evaporation of isocyanates by greatly increasing contact with air. For processes using polymeric MDI and polymeric HDI, these materials will mainly be present in the air as aerosols even if the application process involves spraying of the product or the production of airborne dust. Isocyanates have high odour thresholds above the current ACGIH TLV© and STEL values, therefore, using smell as an indicator of exposure is impractical [ACGIH, 2022].

(a) Aliphatic isocyanates
* **HDI**: Hexamethylene diisocyanate; or 1,6-Diisocyanatehexane (CAS number 822-06-0, MW 168.2)

* **HDI Biuret** (CAS number 97917-21-0, MW 478.6)

* **HDI Uretdione** (MW 336.4)

* **HDI Isocyanurate** (MW 504.7)

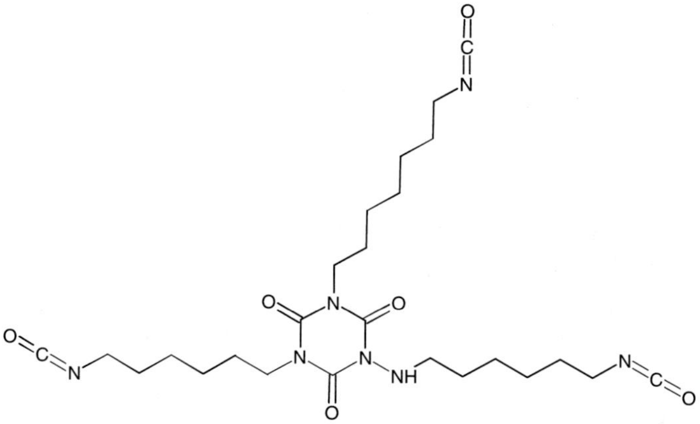

Isocyanates

* **HMDI**: Dicyclohexylmethane 4,4'-diisocyanate; 4,4'-methylenedicyclohexyl diisocyanate; or Methylene bis(4-cyclohexylisocyanate) (CAS number 5124-30-1, MW 262.3).

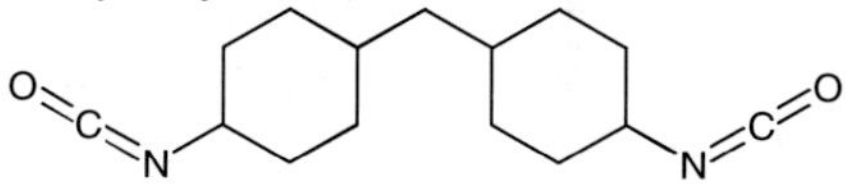

* **IPDI**: Isophorone diisocyanate (CAS number 4098-71-9, MW 222.3)

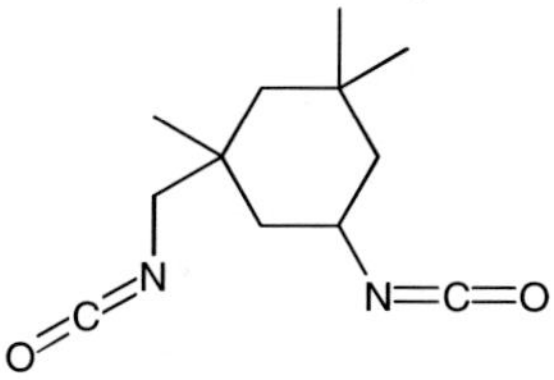

(b) Aromatic isocyanates
* **2,4-TDI**: Toluene-2,4-diisocyanate; or 2,4-Diisocyanatetoluene; (CAS number 584-84-9, MW 174.2)
* **2,6-TDI**: Toluene-2,6-diisocyanate; or 2,6-Diisocyanatetoluene; (CAS number 91-08-7, MW 174.2)

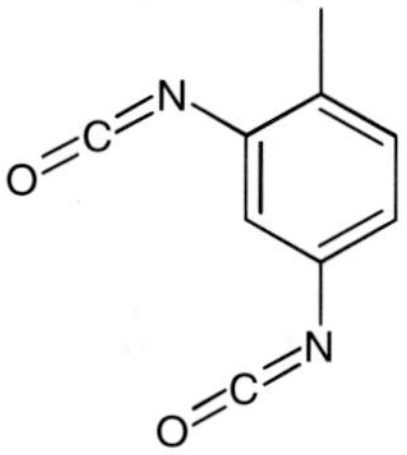

2,4-TDI 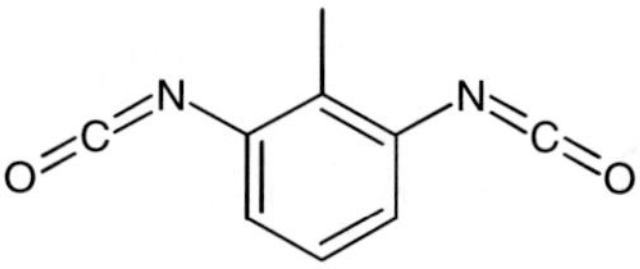   2,6-TDI

Figure 1.1. (Continued).

* **TDI Oligomer**: e.g., TDI Tetraisocyanate (MW 332.3)

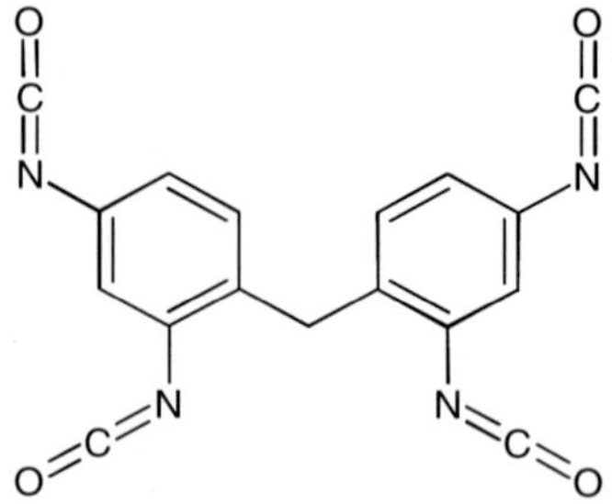

* **MDI**: Methylene diphenyl isocyanate (CAS number 101-68-8, MW 250.2)

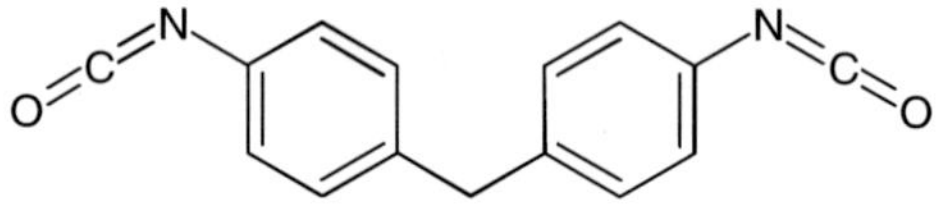

* **MDI Oligomer**:

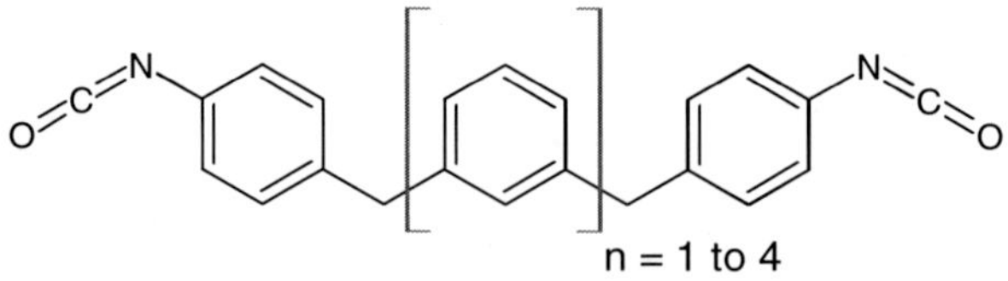

n = 1 to 4

e.g., MDI tetraisocyanate (MW 512.5)

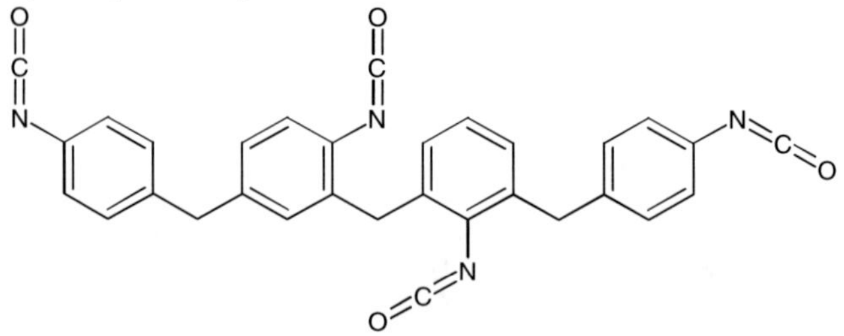

* **Pre-polymer**: e.g., 4,4- MDI polyisocyanate (CAS number 9016-87-9, MW 688.9)

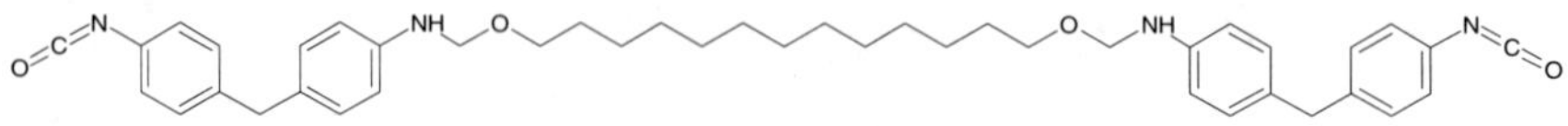

Figure 1.1. Chemical structures of selected isocyanates of major commercial values. (a) Aliphatic isocyanates and (b) Aromatic isocyanates.

1.2. Production and Reactivity

Due to containing the functional group –NCO, isocyanates are highly reactive and unstable compounds.

Isocyanates are usually produced from amines by phosgenation, i.e., treated with phosgene:

$$R-NH_2 + COCl_2 \longrightarrow R-N=C=O + 2HCl$$

These reactions proceed via the intermediary of a caramel chloride. Special precautions are required in the production of isocyanates due to the hazardous nature of phosgene [Six and Richer, 2015].

Another route to isocyanates involves the addition of isocyanic acid to alkenes. Complementarily, alkyl isocyanates form by displacement reactions involving alkyl halides and alkali metal cyanates [Reinhard and Ulrich, 1977].

Isocyanates are electrophiles, and as such they are reactive towards a variety of nucleophiles including alcohols, amines, and even water, having a higher reactivity compared to structurally analogous isothiocyanates [Li et al., 2020]. As isocyanates are highly reactive compounds, there is need for rapid stabilisation after sampling [Henneken 2006], in which isocyanates must be trapped or be stabilised with another reagent to form derivatives during sampling. The reactivity of isocyanates with amines makes amine a better candidate that is applied to sampling airborne isocyanates at workplace. The commonly used agents, or derivatisation agents are 1-(2-methoxypheny)piperazine (1,2-MP or MOPIP), dibutylamine (DBA), etc. Their reactions are demonstrated as below:

Isocyanate + DBA → Isocyanate & DBA derivative

[Reaction scheme: Isocyanate (R-N=C=O) + 1,2-MP (MOPIP) → Isocyanate & 1,2-MP derivative]

Isocyanate   1,2-MP (MOPIP)   Isocyanate & 1,2-MP derivative

As the reaction of isocyanates and amines such as DBA and 1,2-MP undergoes in seconds with a complete conversion, this chemical properties of isocyanates and amines have been widely used in sampling of isocyanates in air [HSE MDHS 25, 2014, Sigma-Aldrich, 2013].

1.3. Common Applications

Isocyanate compounds represent the most important class of heterocumulenes. A heterocumulene is a molecule or ion containing a chain of at least three double bonds between consecutive atoms, in which one or more atoms in the doubly bonded chain is a heteroatom.

Isocyanates chemicals have been found in a wide variety of synthetic applications. These applications include the preparation of amides, esters, peptides, nucleotides, heterocyclic compounds; the identification of amines, alcohols, and nucleic acids; the synthesis of bioactive compounds revealing a wide spectrum of biological activity; the design of effective medicines, herbicides and insecticides; and as chemical intermediates in the production of polyurethane products such as foams, coatings, and elastomers [Bennett, 2017].

Aliphatic isocyanates, such as those based on HDI, are primarily onsite as curing agents in the formation of polyurethane paint systems for automobile refinishing, marine coatings and other high performance coating systems due to their excellent resistance to chemicals and abrasion, and superior weathering characteristics such as gloss and colour retention. Free HDI monomer content of the paint and coating systems range from 0.5% to 1.6% HDI. Aromatic isocyanates include TDI, which is volatile at room temperature and is used in foam manufacture, vanishes and paints, adhesives, surface coatings and the insulation around copper wire used in electronics and liberated during soldering. MDI, which is another aromatic isocyanate, is solid at room temperature and is used in polyurethane foam manufacture, adhesives, binders and elastomers and cores for casting in foundries. A list of the widely used industrial isocyanates and their main uses is in Table 1.1.

Table 1.1. A list of widely used industrial isocyanates and their main uses

Name	Form	Main uses
TDI	Liquid (mix of isomers)	Flexible polyurethane foam production
MDI	Low-melting point solid	Rigid polyurethane foam production
HDI	Liquid	Spray paints, lacquers and car re-finishing
NDI	Solid	Elastomers and synthetic rubbers
IPDI	Liquid	Manufacture of coating and adhesive polymers and polyurethane foams

1.3.1. Manufacturing of Isocyanates

The main process to produce isocyanates is the phosgenation of corresponding diamines. Due to the dangerous properties of two reactants, phosgene and isocyanates themselves, the production processes are carried out under containment in high closed systems [Falcke et al., 2017]. As long as the productions run under normal operating conditions, occupational exposure to isocyanates at this point is generally believed to be low compared with the uses covering the application phases.

1.3.2. Use in Manufacturing of PUs and PU Composite Materials

Production of polyurethane (PU) materials is the major use of isocyanates and has the highest volume. To produce PUs the isocyanates are reacted with macropolyols and/or other polynucleophiles and usually optional additives like catalysts, surfactants, stabilisers, flame retardants, etc. In addition, the polyaddition reaction of isocyanates with the nucleophiles is highly exothermic.

The reactions are typically completed within seconds to up to 30 minutes, whereby the isocyanate groups form urethane bonds with the polyol in the polymer backbone. However, the final curing and posy-curing of PUs, in which exposure to unreacted isocyanates is still possible may take up to 72 hours. Occupational exposure often occur on a regular basis in the manufacture of PU materials and can be frequent. On the other hand, exposure control measures by means of technical controls/measures are often applied at workplaces, so that exposure can be maintained at moderate levels. Note that MDI is the most used isocyanate species for production of PU materials.

1.3.3. Use in Manufacture of Foams

PU foams are generally classified by their elasticity as flexible, semi-flexible, and rigid foams. Foams are also the largest market for PUs and flexible foams are the largest component. MDI and TDI are used in the manufacture of foams. High molecular polyols with two to six hydroxy functionalities produce flexible foams.

Technical control measures to decrease exposure are usually applicable at the mixing unit and the following part of the conveyer belt. At the end of the lines where curing of the slab-stock still takes place are out in the open, exposure to residual isocyanates is extremely possible.

1.3.4. Use in Spray Foam Applications

Spray foam applications is considered as a special circumstance. This is because they are related to particularly high exposure levels, compared with the applications in technically controlled environments (e.g., manufacturing) or where only low mechanic energies are used and therefore no or very low aerosol formation is to be expected (e.g., gluing).

Spray foams are typically two-component rigid foams with one component that is an isocyanate-containing hardener (usually MDI based) and the other component that is a polyol formulation (including catalysts, the blowing agent, and other additives such as flame retardants, surfactants, etc.).

Spray foams are mainly applied for insulation of buildings or industrial installations but can also serve as a speciality packing material for fragile items. This use is particularly challenging in terms of exposure reduction and risk management as aerosol formation during spraying is unavoidable. In addition, spray foam installation is often performed in dynamic workplaces (e.g., at construction sites), which makes technical exposure reduction measures more challenging. When spray foams are used in confined spaces (e.g., insulation of crawl spaces under basement), some technical measures like enclosures or exhaust ventilation might be not achievable at all or to a limited extent. Risk management and exposure reduction therefore is mainly subject to personal protective equipment [Allport et al., 2003].

1.3.5. Use in Coatings

Coatings are often used on surfaces by spraying or by spreading. During these applications, often aerosols are generated and/or splashes happen. It is then often linked to particularly high exposures compared that have uses with no (or minimal) aerosol/droplet formation.

PU coatings can be one-component (one pack) or two-component systems. One-pack paints consisting of free isocyanates are typically high molecular prepolymers of polyols with extra isocyanate groups that underdo a cross link reaction with atmospheric moisture. Two-component systems form the "conventional" PU paints and coatings and are by far the most important systems [Adam et al., 2005]. The cross-linking constituents are polyisocyantes based on TDI, HDI, isophorone diisocyanate (IPDI), MDI, or 4,4-methylenedicyclohexyl diisocyanate (HMDI). The other component of the paint comprises polyols and/or polyamines as well as additives such as pigments, catalysts, and solvents. Both components are mixed instantly before application (preferably in an equimolar ratio). Owing to their outstanding properties (especially high mechanical resistance), PU coatings are the systems of choice for protecting coatings like vehicle finishes and refinish, and in the building sector (floor coatings, anti-corrosion coatings, etc.). Aliphatic isocyanates (especially HDI) are important basic materials for protective and decorative coating systems, especially in motor vehicle repair, where HDI-based spray paints are widely used.

Inhalation exposure to MDI as well as TDI during use of isocyanates is found to be moderately low compared with systems based on the more volatile HDI.

1.3.6. Use in Adhesives

PU adhesives are applied in a wide scope of uses and products ranging from extremely stable and weatherproof woodworking and construction glues to bonding motor vehicle parts (e.g., windshields). The adhesives can be two-component or one-component systems, which themselves can be solvent-based, water-borne (aqueous dispersions), or solvent-free (granulates, dry powders). With respect to potential exposure, it was demonstrated that both the content of isocyanate monomers and the processing temperature have a substantial impact on emissions [Cuno et al., 2015].

Chapter 2

Health and Safety

2.1. Introduction

Isocyanates are used in a wide range of industrial products, including paints, glues and resins. There are potential health effects from isocyanate exposure, including potent respiratory and skin sensitisers and they are a common cause of asthma and allergic contact dermatitis. Isocyanates are essentially a respiratory hazard. They affect the lungs and cause an asthmatic-type reaction and inflammation. As a result, the worker is likely to suffer from the exposure of isocyanates at work. If the workers have continual exposure, some workers will go past a certain point and their lungs will be sensitised. That means if they get even the slightest whiff of an isocyanate they will have a severe asthma-type response and will have problems working at all in that sort of environment. Therefore, the workers who are sensitised will essentially have to stay away from isocyanates and not be able to work in an area where they are present.

There are also potential skin and eye effects because the isocyanates used are liquids. It can cause dermatitis and that is obviously another layer of problem for workers. Certainly, it is an issue affecting the eyes (e.g., stinging) and will be uncomfortable depending on the exposure levels. A range of other adverse health effects are also associated with isocyanate exposure, including cancer. There are some versions that are suspected to be carcinogens.

A study [Kreis et al., 2019] found that occupational lung and skin diseases resulted in a significant economic problem for the patient and the society, although the study claimed there were limitations and substantial differences in their methodology.

The first step for a workplace to go about finding out what their workers' exposure levels to isocyanates are is to look at Safety and Data Sheet (SDS). The SDS tells what is contained in the product, what the concerns are and the potential responses.

The next step is to undertake risk assessment to know what is going on and what controls need to be put in place, ideally higher order controls. The assessment includes finding out how much isocyanate has been exposed to the workers. There are air and biological sampling methods available for quantification.

If the levels of isocyanate exposure are found to have exceeded the standard exposure limit, a range of controls will be considered by the workplace. Where isocyanates are used or unintentionally generated, for example when polyurethanes are heated, it is important that workers' exposures are properly controlled. There are various ways of achieving this, and the way that the isocyanate is used or generated often dictates which control strategy is needed. All exposure controls require maintenance if they are to remain effective, and this chapter provides information on how to achieve this for isocyanates.

2.2. Hazard Statements

The Safe Work Australia [SWA 2015] document "Deemed Diseases in Australia" reviews the latest scientific evidence on the causal link between diseases and occupational exposures. It is determined that the key disease caused by isocyanates was occupational asthma. The SWA [SWA 2021] Hazardous Substance Information System (HSIS) provides classifications on hazard statements for isocyanates (Table 2.1).

Table 2.1. Hazard statements for isocyanates in HSIS

Health Hazard Statement	Isocyanate Type
H 302 (Harmful if swallowed)	HDI
H 314 (Causes severe skin burns and eye damage)	HDI
H 315 (Causes skin irritation)	2,4-TDI, MDI, IPDI & HMDI
H 317 (May cause an allergic skin reaction)	2,4-TDI, HDI, MDI, IPDI & HMDI
H 319 (Causes serious eye irritation)	2,4-TDI, MDI, IPDI & HMDI
H 330 (Fatal if inhaled)	HDI, 2,4-TDI & MDI
H 331 (Toxic if inhaled)	IPDI & HMDI
H 334 (May cause allergy or asthma symptoms)	2,4-TDI
H 335 (May cause respiratory irritation)	2,4-TDI, MDI, IPDI & HMDI
H 351 (Suspected of causing cancer)	2,4-TDI, MDI
H 372 (Causes damage to organs through inhalation)	HDI, MDI

2.3. Exposure Routes

Isocyanate exposure generally occurs through inhalation and/or dermal routes. Depending on the isocyanate type and the application method, there may be significant exposure potential from either, or both, of these routes and the risk management approach should be considered.

Inhalation exposure can occur when isocyanates are present in the workplace air, either as a vapour or an aerosol. In some instances, airborne isocyanates can be present in both of these forms simultaneously.

Vapours can be generated from passive processes by evaporation, and the volatility of the isocyanate chemicals will influence the degree of airborne vapour which it generates. Evaporation will increase as the process temperature increases, and so the heating of isocyanates will increase vapour levels in air. Liquid isocyanates are often very viscous at ambient temperature and are usually heated to help them flow better for making them easier to handle. This will increase the rate of isocyanate vapour generation. Similarly, the isocyanate-polyol reaction which takes place to form a polyurethane is highly exothermic, generating a lot of heat. As a result, this will increase vapour generation, even if no external heat is added to the process.

Aerosols can be generated by deliberate means, such as spraying, or inadvertently when isocyanate materials are mechanically agitated or vigorously disturbed. For example, fine aerosol particles will be generated when liquids are brush applied or poured from one container to another. However, the amount of aerosol generated in this way will usually be much lower than from spraying processes. Where solid isocyanates are handled, there is potential for airborne dust to be generated.

Dermal (skin) exposure can occur wherever there is potential for workers' skin to come into contact with isocyanate materials. The main mechanisms by which dermal exposure to isocyanates occur are:

- Direct contact with workers' skin;
- Deposition of aerosol from the air onto workers' skin;
- Splashing, during pouring or mixing activities;
- Handling contaminated items such as tools or used personal protective equipment (PPE);
- Contact with contaminated surfaces, such as control panels or process plant, such as during maintenance.

2.4. Risk Management

Given the toxicity of isocyanates, it is important to control worker exposures to these chemicals wherever they are used or generated. A thorough risk assessment is part of the process of achieving adequate control. This will allow an appropriate exposure control strategy to be defined and implemented. Risk assessment for dangerous substances is a legal requirement. The hierarchy of control should be observed when designing exposure control strategies.

Occupational exposure limits (OELs) for isocyanates exist in various countries but these do not necessarily represent safe levels of exposure. In the case of isocyanates, exposures should be controlled to be reduced to a minimum. This is because some individuals are more susceptible to sensitisation effects than others, and even exposures to substantially low OELs can lead to serious health effects.

In terms of respiratory effects, processes which generate high airborne levels of isocyanates, such as spray application, carry the greatest risk. It is important to emphasise that all airborne isocyanates, whether they are monomeric or polymeric, in either aerosol or vapour phase, are harmful. Even where airborne levels are likely to be very low, such as brush or roller application of low volatility polymeric isocyanates, the potential for skin effects still exists and must be taken into consideration when developing an exposure control strategy.

2.4.1. Exposure Controls

Precautionary statements for prevention of exposure or contact with individual isocyanates available from SDS should be followed. Controls should focus on prevention of respiratory and skin exposure. It is considered very important that people using these compounds understand the associated health hazards, especially the risk of sensitisation and are trained in using the controls effectively. Inappropriate selection and use of respirators and gloves contribute greatly to isocyanate exposure. For example, air purifying respirators with a protection factor of 25 or greater are required to protect against isocyanate exposures during spray painting [Reeb-Whitaker et al., 2012].

2.4.1.1. Elimination/Substitution

According to the principles of good occupational hygiene practice, and the hierarchy of control (Figure 2.1), elimination of a hazard, or substitution with a less hazardous material or a less hazardous application technique is a preferable control option to solutions based on engineering controls and PPE. Control solutions based on substitution include:

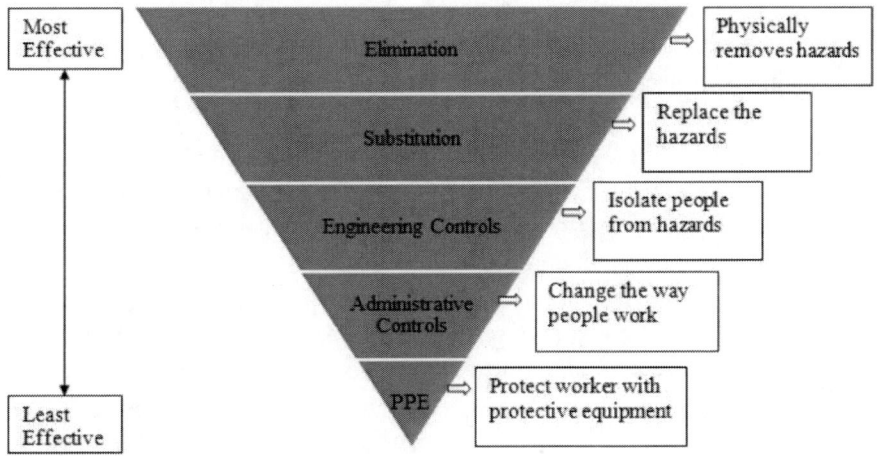

Figure 2.1. A diagram of hierarchy of controls.

It is possible to replace isocyanate-based paints with other less hazardous products which can still achieve acceptable quality and durability of finish. To use water-based paints is the current trend in the industry. However, "water-based" does not mean "isocyanates-free", just that it is emulsion based and has reduced levels of solvents. The less solvent content in spray paints help reduce isocyanate evaporation during spray painting.

Another technique is the use of pre-polymeric isocyanates rather than monomers. For decades now, the amount of free monomeric isocyanate has been greatly reduced from 0.5% to 0.1%. In this instance, although the isocyanate is still present, it is in a less volatile form and so the potential for vapour generation is reduced. To further reduce occupational exposure to isocyanates, a restriction on products containing more than 0.1% by weight of isocyanates was recently adopted by the EU's REACH Regulation in 2016 [Rother and Schluter, 2021].

The adoption of various application techniques helps to lower process emissions. The use of brush or roller application for paints, instead of spraying, significantly reduces the potential for inhalation exposure.

2.4.1.2. Engineering Control

Where substitution of isocyanate materials at the workplace is not possible, engineering control solutions based on separating the worker from the exposure source are seen as the next best option. Engineering controls can take various forms, with the following being most relevant for controlling isocyanate exposures:

- *Containment*: This would include the use of sealed handling systems for transferring bulk material from storage tanks to the point of use, or the use of lids on containers when not in use, to prevent vapour emission into the workroom.
- *Process modification*: High volume low pressure (HVLP) spray guns are available for spraying isocyanate paints. These reduce the amount of paint used and minimise aerosol generation.
- *Local Exhaust Ventilation (LEV)*: This would include the use of fume cupboards and ventilated cabinets for the storage and handling of small to medium quantities of isocyanates and the use of ventilated spray booths for the application of 2 pack paints in the motor vehicle repair (MVR) industry.
- *Segregation*: In some situations it may not be possible to apply LEV effectively to control exposure. In such instances, segregating the workplace to contain the isocyanate in designated, clearly signed areas will reduce the spread of contamination and protect workers who are not directly involved in the process.
- *Safe working distance*: The use of tools to increase the distance between the worker and the exposure source can significantly reduce dermal and inhalation exposure. Examples would include the use of long handled rollers for the smoothing of isocyanate flooring and the use of a spatula rather than a gloved hand to remove viscous isocyanates from tins.

2.4.1.3. Personal Protective Equipment

PPE is generally seen as a less reliable exposure control than those discussed above and should be used as the last resort only. However, PPE still has a part to play and there may be processes with a high potential for exposure, even after the implementation of engineering controls, where PPE is the only means of achieving adequate control. The following issues are of specific relevance to isocyanates.

- Chemical protective gloves should be used as splash protection only, processes should not be designed such that gloves are used as a primary barrier against direct contact with isocyanates or isocyanate contaminated work equipment. Gloves should be selected which offer the appropriate level of chemical protection whilst also taking into consideration other factors such as the need for thermal protection or manual dexterity.
- Work overalls and oversuits should provide whole body coverage and not leave susceptible body parts, such as forearms, open to exposure. Disposable coveralls may offer a better solution than re-usable garments which can become heavily contaminated over time, and potentially act as an additional exposure source.
- Respiratory protective equipment (RPE) must be selected taking into account the 'control challenge' (i.e., airborne concentrations of isocyanate outside the RPE) and usage factors such as the length of time for which it will be worn and the need for other PPE, such as eye protection. Airborne isocyanates can be present in the atmosphere at harmful levels and not be detectable by smell, hence it would not be immediately obvious to the wearer if a filtering respirator were to fail. For this reason, the use of air supplied RPE is generally the preferred option for processes with high potential for inhalation exposure. This would apply to all manual spraying processes, such as paint spraying or the application of polyurethane foam insulation. Filtering respirators may be acceptable for processes with lower airborne emissions. Exposure monitoring can play a key role in RPE selection. If RPE is selected which requires a good seal to the workers face for effective operation, it is important that the RPE fits the worker correctly. Face fit testing is required to ensure this.

In all cases PPE must be selected, used, stored and maintained correctly in order to obtain maximum protection.

2.4.1.4. The Practicalities of Achieving Adequate Control
It is almost always the case that a practical, effective exposure control strategy will use a combination of exposure controls. In designing a control strategy, all exposure routes should be considered and the hierarchy of control applied for each exposure route. Processes should be designed to limit the potential for workers to come into contact with isocyanates. PPE for controlling dermal exposure should be provided for splash protection and not as a primary barrier against direct contact with isocyanates and heavily contaminated work equipment.

LEV will often be a necessary part of achieving control and preventing the spread of airborne contamination into areas occupied by other workers not directly involved with the isocyanate process. However, this control approach can fail due to poor design, incorrect use or inadequate maintenance. The design and implementation of an effective LEV system requires the specialist expertise of ventilation engineers and occupational hygienists. It is vital to establish that the system provides adequate control when it is commissioned.

For some processes involving spray application of isocyanates, LEV systems alone cannot provide adequate control of inhalation exposure, even where they are well designed and properly used. RPE will also be required in these circumstances [White et al., 2006]. In MVR, the role of the ventilated booth is to reduce the airborne isocyanate levels as far as possible during spraying, to remove airborne isocyanate from the spray space as quickly as possible after spraying, and to contain the airborne contamination within the spray space to prevent other workers being exposed. It is essential to consider that all spray booths take time to clear airborne isocyanates after spraying is complete. Even when the visible spray has cleared, which usually happens quite quickly, dangerously high levels of airborne isocyanate can remain for several minutes. It is common practice amongst spray painters to lift the visor of full face RPE immediately after spraying to inspect the paint finish. This results in peaks of very high inhalation exposure and adds significantly to the risk of developing asthma. The manual cleaning of spray guns can also give rise to high isocyanate exposures, in addition to the cleaning solvents. Spray guns should not be cleaned in the open workshop or paint mixing room.

Wherever possible exposure controls should be designed and built into the process. It is always more difficult to achieve adequate control when measures are retro fitted to existing plant and machinery.

All exposure controls require maintenance if they are to offer sustained exposure control. LEV systems should be tested frequently, and filters changed at recommended intervals. PPE requires appropriate checking and maintenance. Where air fed RPE is used it is important to ensure that the breathing air is clean and supplied at an adequate flow rate and pressure. This also applies to 'software' controls, where regular refresher training of workers is appropriate.

2.4.2. Exposure Standards

The development of OELs is thought to have begun with reports published in 1883 by Max Gruber, a German scientist who studied the effects of carbon monoxide at varying air concentrations by exposing both himself and laboratory animals [Cook, 1987; Paustenbach 1998]. The first systematic collection of "modern" OELs was developed in 1946 by The American Conference of Governmental Industrial Hygienist (ACGIH) subcommittee, which had been directed to derive and maintain such a system of exposure limits. In 1956, the term Threshold Limit Value (TLV) was adopted in lieu of the term Maximal Allowable Concentration.

2.4.2.1. Airborne Monitoring

Current OELs for the acceptable levels of isocyanates range among different countries.

Two approaches are currently used to express OELs for isocyanates levels in air. The most common approach is to describe the OEL for individual isocyanates as either parts per million (ppm) -or micrograms per cubic meter of air ($\mu g/m^3$).

The second approach expresses the OEL in terms of total number of NCO groups within an isocyanate mixture, rather than quantifying each individual species. This OEL is expressed as the mass of total NCO groups or as "μg NCO m^{-3}" and may be referred to as the Total Reactive Isocyanate Group (TRIG).

A summary from the USA and UK of existing airborne OELs for isocyanates is presented in Table 2.2 [Streicher et al., 2000]. The majority of these OELs are for diisocyanate monomers and only a few exist for polyisocyanates, despite the known human adverse health effects of polyisocyanate exposure. The Occupational Safety and Health Administration (OSHA) has ceiling Permissible Exposure Limits (PELs) for TDI and MDI monomers, but no 8-hr-time weighted average (TWA) standard for isocyanates or polyisocyanates. The National Institutes for Occupational Safety and Health (NIOSH) has ceiling and full-shift TWA recommended exposure limits (RELs) for several diisocyanate monomers, but none for polyisocyanates. The ACGIH has primarily full-shift TWA threshold limit values (TLVs) for a variety of monomers with a short-term exposure limit (STEL) set only for TDI monomer. ACHIH has no polyisocyanaye TLVs. The OSHA, ACGIH, and NIOSH OELs for isocyanate monomers are all based on the monomer mass concentration.

Table 2.2. Current USA (OSHA, NIOSH, ACGIH) and UK-HSE Occupational Exposure Limits (OEL) ($\mu g/m^3$ air) for Isocyanates

Isocyanate species	OSHA PEL		NIOSH REL		ACGIH TLV		UK-HSE OEL	
	TWA 8-hr	Ceiling	TWA 10-hr	Ceiling 10 min	TWA 8-hr	STEL 15 min	TWA 8-hr	Ceiling 10 min
TDI	-	140 (68)	CA-LFG[a]	-	36 (17)	140 (68)		
MDI	-	200 (67)	50 (17)	200 (67)	51 (17)	-		
NDI	-	-	40 (16)	170 (68)	-	-		
HDI	-	-	35 (18)	140 (70)	34 (17)	-		
IPDI	-	-	45 (17)	180 (68)	45 (17)	-		
HMDI			-	110 (35)	54 (17)	-		
Total NCO[b]	-	-	-	-	-	-	(20)	(70)

Bracketed values represent the equivalent standard in μg NCO/m^3.
[a] NIOSH considers TDI to be an occupational carcinogen (CA) and recommends that exposures be reduced to the lowest feasible concentration (LFG).
[b] Total reactive isocyanate group in μg NCO group/m^3. The standard applies to all isocyanate species (monomers, polyisocyanates, and their mixtures) regardless of their origin.

The United Kingdom Health and Safety Executive (UK-HSE) has taken a very different approach to regulating isocyanate using total NCO as the exposure metric. This approach combines all monomers and polyisocyanates into a single total isocyanate standard which is expressed as micrograms NCO group/m^3. The UK-HSE sets the maximum exposure limits at 20 μg NCO/m^3 for the full shift and 70 μg NCO/m^3 for a 15-minute short-term exposure limit (STEL) [HSE 1999]. The Australian National Occupational Safety and Health Commission (NOSHC) has also adopted the UK-HSE maximum exposure limits for isocyanates [NOHSC 1995].

All of these standards are expressed either as the pure product mass concentration for isocyanate-specific OELs (USA), or as a non-specific NCO mass concentration (UK). Unlike isocyanate-specific OELs for monomers and HDI polyisocyanate, the UK total NCO standards are a sum of monomer and prepolymeric isocyanate group content.

2.4.2.2. Biological Monitoring

Table 2.3 shows values that should be used as a guide for assessing exposure to isocyanates when urine analysis for isocyanate metabolites is performed.

Table 2.3. Reference values for assessing biological exposure to isocyanates

Biological level	Source
1 μmol of isocyanate-derived diamine/mol creatinine in urine	BMGV from HSE
5 μg TDA/g creatinine and 15 μg HDA/g creatinine in urine	BAT from DFG
10 μg MDA/L (50 nmol/L; 6 μmol MDA/mol Creatinine) in urine	BLW from DFG
5 μg TDA/g creatinine and 15 μg HDA/g creatinine in urine	BEI from ACGIH

The UK HSE (2020) has a Biological Monitoring Guidance Value (BMGV) for isocyanates. It is based on a urine sample taken at the end of exposure and is measured for the corresponding diisocyanate diamine. The BMGV is based on 'good occupational hygiene practice' and was set at the 90th percentile of results (1 μmol/mol creatinine) from a dataset where exposure controls were deemed to be adequate. The urine test can check exposures for at least the four main isocyanates in use (HDI, IPDI, TDI & MDI) so the test can be helpful in a wide range of industries using isocyanates (polyurethane moulding, foam blowing, use of adhesives etc.) [Jones, 2019].

The ACGIH [AIGIH 2022] has a Biological Exposure Index (BEI) for TDI (2,4- & 2,6-isomers) exposures of 5 μg/g creatinine (3 μmol/mol creatinine) of toluene diamine in urine; and a BEI for HDI of 15 μg/g creatinine (10 μmol/mol creatinine) of 1,6-hexane diamine, collected at the end of shift.

The German research institute, Deutsche Forschungsgemeinschaft (DFG), have listed the biological tolerance values (BAT - Biologische Arbeitsstoff Toleranzwerte) for HDI exposures of 15 μg/g creatinine (10 μmol/mol creatinine) of 1,6-hexane diamine; and for TDI (2,4- & 2,6-isomers) exposures of 5 μg/g creatinine (3 μmol/mol creatinine) of the sum of 2,4 & 2,6 toluene diamine isomers in urine collected at the end of exposure or shift. They have listed a biological guidance value (BLW - Biologische Leit-Werte) value of 10 μg/L (50 nmol/L; 6 μmol/mol creatinine) for MDI measured as 4,4'-Diaminodiphenyl methane in urine at the end of exposure or shift [DFG 2022].

There is a substantial body of work demonstrating the utility of biological monitoring as a tool to assess exposure and the efficacy of controls, including how it can be used in assessing exposure to isocyanates in the workplace. Non-health based biological monitoring guidance values are also available to help target when and where further action is required. Occupational hygienists will need to use their knowledge and experience to determine the relative contributions of different routes of exposure and how controls can be improved to reduce the risk of ill health [Cocker, 2011].

2.4.3. Regulation

United States
The OSHA is the regulatory body covering worker safety. OSHA puts forth Permissible Exposure Limit (PEL) 20 ppb for MDI and detailed technical guidance on exposure assessment [NMCPHC 2018].

The NIOSH is the agency responsible for providing the research and recommendations regarding workplace safety, while OSHA is more of an enforcement body. NIOSH is responsible for producing the science that can result in RELs, which can be lower than the PEL. OSHA is tasked with enforcement and defending the PELs. In 1992, when OSHA reduced the PEL for TDI to the NIOSH REL, the PEL reduction was challenged in court, and the reduction was reversed [NIOSH 1996].

The Environmental Protection Agency (EPA) is also involved in the regulation of isocyanates with regard to the environment and also non-worker persons that might be exposed [USEPA 2015].

The ACGIH is a non-government organization that publishes guidance known as threshold limit values (TLV) [NIOSH 1996] for chemicals based research as constant work exposure level without ill-effect. The TLV is not an OSHA-enforceable value, unless the PEL is the same.

European Union
The European Chemicals Agency (ECHA) provides regulatory oversight of chemicals used within the European Union [ECHA 2018]. ECHA has been implementing policy aimed at limiting worker exposure through elimination by lower allowable concentrations in products and mandatory worker training, as an administrative control [Vincentz 2018]. Within the European Union, many nations set their own occupational exposure limits for isocyanates.

International Groups
The United Nations, through the World Health Organization (WHO) together with the International Labour Organization (ILO) and United Nations Environment Programme (UNEP), collaborate on the International Programme on Chemical Safety (IPCS) to publish summary documents on

chemicals. The IPCS published one such document in 2000 summarizing the status of scientific knowledge on MDI [Sekizawa and Greenberg 2000].

The International Agency for Research on Cancer (IARC) evaluates the hazard data on chemicals and assigns a rating on the risk of carcinogenesis. In the case of TDI, the final evaluation is possibly carcinogenic to humans (Group 2B) [IARC 71-37]. For MDI, the final evaluation is not classifiable as to its carcinogenicity to humans (Group 3) [IARC 71-47].

The International Isocyanate Institute (III) is an international industry consortium that seeks to promote the safe utilization of isocyanates by disseminating best practices [III 2018].

2.4.4. Exposure Monitoring

Exposure monitoring can play a key part in the risk management approach to handling isocyanates [Creely et al., 2006]. This can be broadly segregated into two areas, air sampling and biological monitoring.

2.4.4.1. Air Sampling
From an occupational hygiene viewpoint, the most common and useful form of air sampling is personal monitoring. This allows the best estimation of worker exposure, and can be an essential element in ascertaining the adequacy of control and informing RPE selection. The measurement of airborne isocyanates is complex and requires specialist expertise [White 2006a and White et al., 2012]. Some measurement methods only quantify certain isocyanate species, most commonly monomers. Industrial isocyanate preparations are frequently a mixture of pre-polymers, all of which are harmful to health. Other techniques are only applicable to vapour phase or particulate phase airborne isocyanate. To be of value to the risk assessment process, the measurement method must identify and quantify all isocyanates in monomeric and polymeric forms, whether in the vapour phase or present as airborne particulate. In particular, methods which only quantify monomeric isocyanates can grossly underestimate exposure, and give an impression that the risk is low when harmful levels of airborne isocyanate are present. Where possible, measurement methodology which is accredited by a reputable organisation should be employed. A number of isocyanate measurement methods have been developed and published by NIOSH, OSHA, HSE, DFG, and some methods have ISO accreditation [ISO 17734-1, 17736, 17735, & 16702].

2.4.4.2. Biological Monitoring

Biological monitoring offers a useful approach to exposure assessment [Cocker, 2007] and can provide a reliable indication of recent occupational exposure. Biological monitoring can be cheaper and easier to administer than air sampling, and can provide information on total exposure by all routes, and on the efficacy of PPE in controlling exposure. Test results above the BMGV indicate the failure of exposure controls which should then be investigated, and effective action taken to ensure they are fully implemented. Certain amines which are used with isocyanates in some industrial processes can interfere with the biological monitoring method. Repeat samples should be taken to check that controls are working and preventing further exposure. Where it is required, this urine sampling should be carried out at least yearly. For new employees, a sample should be taken during the first few months to show that the controls and working practices are providing protection.

2.4.5. Health Surveillance

Health surveillance plays a key part in the risk management approach for isocyanates [Mackie, 2008]. Regular, targeted surveillance by a competent individual can identify the early stages of skin and respiratory disease, and hence allow interventions on an individual and company wide basis to be made. Urine testing for isocyanates only checks whether the worker has been exposed, not whether their health has been affected.

Occupational health is concerned with the effects to the health of the individual from their workplace and the effects that their health may have on their work. Health surveillance and health monitoring offer tools to identify work-related disease or ill health to help minimise the effects and health risks.

Risk-based health surveillance involves specific health assessments or medical tests that can measure the degree of damage done to an employee's health. As different chemicals cause specific health affects it is important to obtain specialist advice from an occupational hygienist, occupational physician or clinical toxicologist before implementing any health surveillance program.

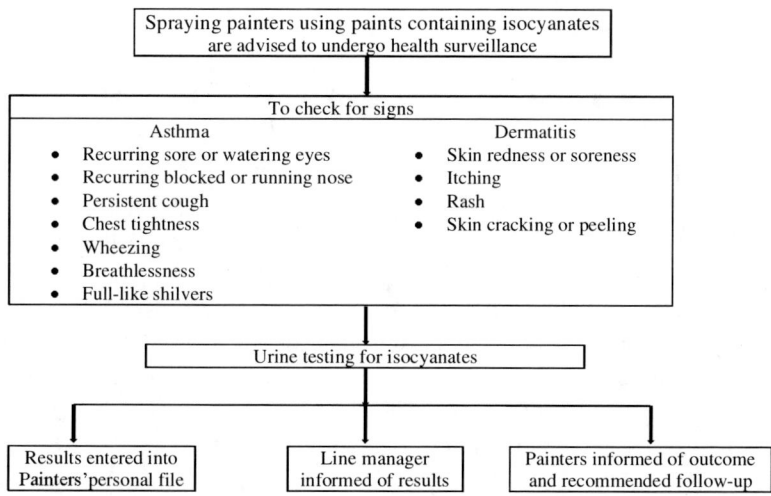

Figure 2.2. A simplified flow chart of health surveillance for the spray painters using paints containing isocyanates.

Risk-based health surveillance, which can incorporate biological monitoring as part of the procedures, assesses possible health effects that may arise if occupational exposures exceed accepted or adopted exposure standards. This assessment is recommended annually for employees at risk of significant exposure in their workplace. This involves: (i) identifying the source and method of exposure; (ii) measuring atmospheric and surface concentrations; and (iii) reviewing the efficacy of control measures. If measured biological levels reach or exceed recommended action levels, a suitable and sufficient health assessment by a competent person is indicated. Follow up testing is recommended within a specified time that depends on the biological half-life of the particular chemical. A medical check-up is required when follow-up testing confirms the level remains above the exposure standards. At this time, additional biological monitoring may be requested, which may involve analysis to detect any early biochemical effects.

A competent person to carry out the above assessment may be an occupational physician or clinical toxicologist with experience in assessing and diagnosing occupational diseases associated with hazardous substance exposures. Depending on the types of health effects that may be caused by the particular substance, individuals may be referred for other medical tests to assess potential biochemical or neurological effects. A simplified flow chart of health surveillance for spraying painters using isocyanate paints is shown in Figure 2.2.

2.5. Conclusion

Isocyanates are important and useful industrial chemicals, with wide ranging applications. However, they have the potential to cause a range of serious health effects, and a rigorous and robust exposure control strategy must be employed wherever isocyanates are used. The specialist skills of a professional occupational hygienist may be needed to ensure that all risks are adequately controlled.

Given the complex aspects of isocyanates toxicity and exposure assessment, rather than depend on an airborne regulatory exposure limit, it would be in the best interest of all stakeholders to have an industrial-specific guidance/best practice approach. Such approaches already exist, including the program described by Gannon et al., 2005, which has the goals of prevention, early detection, and mitigation of effect of key endpoints, especially asthma and a lesser degree dermatitis, in worker who are occupational exposed, or potentially exposed, to isocyanates and products containing isocyanates. Training of workers in the correct use of isocyanate exposure controls is of paramount importance.

With regard to the data for inhalation exposure it has to be kept in mind that measurement of airborne isocyanates is technically challenging and may underestimate actual exposure levels. In addition, peak exposures to isocyanates are particularly difficult to detect, which can also lead to an underestimation of exposure.

To address the risks of occupational asthma caused by isocyanates, the German competent authority for REACH has proposed a restriction of products containing more than 0.1% by weight of isocyanates (individually and in combination) under the EU's REACH Regulation in 2016. The restriction was recently published in the EU Official Journal [European Commission, 2020] and will apply after a transitional period of 3 years from 24 August 2023. Isocyanates are defined therein as 'O=C=N–R–N=C=O, with R an aliphatic or aromatic hydrocarbon unit of unspecified length'. This definition should also apply to oligomers/prepolymers as long as they have two terminal NCO units. It is supposed that this will lead to increased substitution efforts to safer products, i.e., products containing less than 0.1% (w/w) of isocyanates.

However, a derogation from this ban can be made if industrial and professional users receive an obligatory standardized training on good working practices and risk management. Work training has been shown to be an effective measure to reduce occupational exposure to isocyanates [Jones et al., 2019] and the training required by the restriction aims to improve compliance and make working with isocyanates safer.

It is found that the future of OELs of isocyanates face a number of important barriers. Perhaps the most important one to developing OELs of isocyanates and their oligomers is lack of data, and in particular, data that are relevant to human exposure in occupational settings. Another important barrier to the on-going relevance of OELs is lack of systematic approaches for their development, selection, and application, especially in the contexts of missing data and global harmonisation. While never perfect, OELs will and should always be an important and essential tool for anticipating, recognising and controlling workplace hazards such as isocyanates and their relevant oligomers.

Chapter 3

Laboratory Analytical Methods

3.1. Introduction

Many modern analytical instruments have been applied at laboratories to analyse the isocyanates derivatives and isocyanates metabolites. These instruments include gas chromatography (GC) and liquid chromatography (LC) for separation and either of them is coupled with flame ionisation detector (FID), electrochemical detector (ECD) and mass spectrometer (MS) for confirmation and quantitation. Generally, both GC and LC are efficient, highly selective, and widely applicable for the analysis of isocyanate derivatives and metabolites. But depending on the properties of these compounds, LC has the advantage for separating non-volatile or thermally unstable compounds. In terms of application of GC/MS and LC/MS, there was a long delay in applying LC/MS due to the difficulties involved with coupling LC to MS. Since the 1970s various LC-MS interfaces have been developed, but it was only after the launch of atmospheric-pressure interfaces, electrospray ionisation (ESI), atmospheric-pressure chemical ionisation (APCI), and atmospheric pressure photo-ionisation (APPI) that LC-MS began to be a robust alternative to GC/MS methods [Skoog et al., 2017]. Figure 3.1 shows the relationship between the molecular mass range and the polarities of analytes that can be analysed by GC/MS and different LC/MS interface techniques. As can be seen, ESI is the most universal of these interfaces and has become the "golden-standard" of LC/MS today.

Reliable analytical methods are required, and analytical chemists have had to contend with not only isocyanates derivatives from air sampling but also their metabolites from biological monitoring, which must be determined at very low concentration levels in complex matrices. Undoubtedly, optimised chromatographic methods have had to be employed, and compliance with mass spectrometric techniques is compulsory to satisfy the sensitivity and selectivity requirements and confirm the identities of compounds detected in this type of analysis.

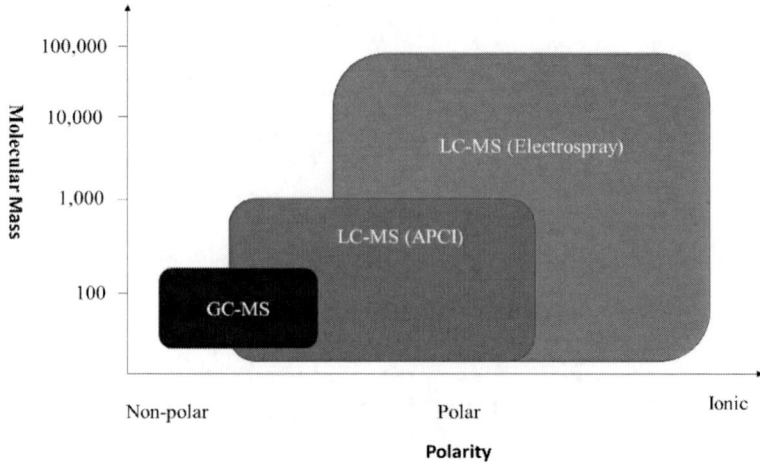

Figure 3.1. Relation of the molecular mass range and the polarity of analytes analysable by GC-MS and LC-MS interface techniques (APCI and ESI).

A vital component of sampling and analytical methods is a sound quality assurance/control program. The programs are typically comprised of multiple testing procedures that easily allow the detection of systematic failures in the methodology. These testing method procedures can include proficiency testing to ensure accuracy as measured against a known reference material, repeat measurements of known reference materials to confirm the validity of an analytical run and to measure analytical precision, "round robin" studies to confirm reproducible measurement values among laboratories analysing for isocyanates and/or metabolites, regular verification of instrument calibration by analysing "blank" samples, and cross validations to ensure that multiple analysts and instruments obtain similar analytical values.

As isocyanates are highly reactive compounds, there is a need for rapid stabilisation after sampling [Henneken, 2006]. Due to the reactivity of isocyanates in air, they must be trapped or stabilised with another reagent to form derivatives during sampling. As a result, isocyanates derivatives are analysed by LC because they are non-volatile. On the other hand, isocyanates metabolites are not suitable for direct analysis by either LC or GC. These metabolites also need derivatisation and then they can be analysed by LC or GC [Williams et al.,1999, Marand et al., 2004]. Some of the common techniques used to analyse isocyanate derivatives and metabolites are outlined below.

3.2. Sample Preparation

Samples subject to analysis are very rarely in a form ready for acquiring the required data. They are usually a complex mixture where the target compound or analyte is present at relatively low levels in relation to the remaining sample constituents. Although some methods can be used to directly analyse a sample, such as "dilute and shoot", they rely on the capability of the analytical system to discriminate the target analyte from the rest of the sample. As explained later in the following sections of the Chapter, the combination of LC with MS provides an analytical technique with a high capability to discriminate between different molecules. Yet, even with this capability, the vast majority of analyses require greater clean-up or concentration of the sample prior to the use of LC-MS in order to achieve the selectivity, sensitivity and robustness required by routine analytical applications.

There are two commonly used sample clean-up methods. They are liquid-liquid extraction (LLE) and solid phase extraction (SPE).

The LLE method is a relatively simple and quick wet chemistry technique based on the solubility of an analyte between two immiscible solvents, where the target analyte passes from its solvent of origin into a "polarity compatible" solvent in which it is more soluble. In the case of a highly non-polar analyte, contained in an aqueous biological matrix such as urine, the analyte will partition into the added immiscible non-polar solvent.

The SPE technique, which is commonly used in both environmental and clinical applications, uses a solid stationary phase sorbent (normally contained in a cartridge) to clean-up and/or concentrate sample prior to analysis. There is a wide range of sorbent chemistries available that are typically surface-modified silica supports, providing great selectivity to strategically retain either the target analyte or interferences present in the sample. For trace analysis, SPE is generally used to selectively isolate and concentrate a known target analyte within the sample.

These two methods have advantages and drawbacks of their own. LLE has a simple operation and uses simple apparatus. But the process is tedious. The method needs to use large volumes of solvents of high purity, which can increase environmental pollution. The enrichment factor of the analyte is often small, and the selectivity is low. The formation of emulsions during operation is often difficult to break. There are problems with handling samples of large volumes.

On the other hand, the SPE method has possibility of storage of enriched analytes on the solid sorbent. The low recoveries of the analytes are possible due to interactions between the sorbent and the matrix or sorbent bed breakthrough.

The currently used method for determination of amines in biological samples as markers of exposure to the amines or corresponding isocyanates involves a sample preparation for the instrumental analysis. The multiple work-up procedures are briefly described below. The urine samples are hydrolysed first, and the amines are extracted into toluene via a liquid-liquid extraction approach. A derivatising agent is added into the toluene phases. The phases containing the amide derivatives are subsequently transferred to vials and then analysed using GC-MS [Williams et al.,1999], or LC-MS [Marand et al., 2004], which will be discussed in detail in the next section.

Fortunately, the sample preparation for analysis of isocyanates in air is relatively easy. Isocyanates in air are sampled by collecting them onto impregnated filters with a derivatising agent and/or impingers containing a derivatising agent solution. The isocyanates react to form urea derivatives and are trapped onto the filters and/or impinger solution. The isocyanate derivatives are relatively stable. At the laboratory, the isocyanate derivatives on filter are desorbed with solvent and then measured by LC. The isocyanate derivatives in the impinger solution are evaporated to dryness, and the dry residues are dissolved with a solvent after dryness, and then measured by LC as well.

3.3. Analytical Techniques

3.3.1. Gas Chromatography

Gas chromatography is a technique for separating mixtures whose components are volatile or can be made so. The separation takes inside an oven which is a capillary column where the separation takes place. A typical capillary column may be 25 meters long with an internal diameter of 250 µm. It is often made of silica. The inside is coated with liquid stationary phase. An inert gas such as helium carries the sample mixtures through capillary. Parts of the sample will show great affinity to stationary phase and travel more slowly. Over the 25 metres, the components of mixtures become separated along the capillary tube. At the end of capillary, the separated components are carried into through a detector such as an FID or MS. Each peak on chromatogram represents the component in the mixture, which are separated on capillary column and are detected in FID or MS. A schematic diagram of Gas chromatograph is shown in Figure 3.2.

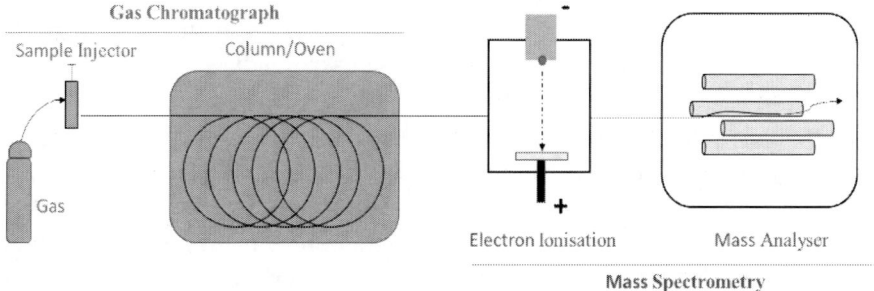

Figure 3.2. Schematic diagram of Gas chromatograph-Mass Spectrometry.

3.3.2. Flame Ionisation Detection

The operation of the FID is based on the detection of ions formed during combustion of organic compounds in a hydrogen flame. The generation of these ions is proportional to the concentration of organic species in the sample gas stream.

Flame ionization detectors are used very widely in gas chromatography because of several advantages such as cost, low maintenance requirements, rugged construction, linearity and detection ranges. FIDs can measure organic substance concentration at low (ng/L) and very high levels, having a linear response range of mg/L. However, flame ionization detectors have many disadvantages such as a lack of selectivity and identification. For example, the FID has no way to identify them if the two molecules elute at the same retention time. This limits the application of FID in analytical laboratories.

3.3.3. Mass Spectrometer

The GC-MS is composed of two major building blocks: the gas chromatograph and the mass spectrometer. The gas chromatograph separates the molecules in the mixtures. The molecules are retained and then elute (come off) from the gas chromatography at different times (called the retention time), and this allows the mass spectrometer downstream to capture, ionize, accelerate, deflect, and detect the ionized molecules separately. The mass spectrometer does this by breaking each molecule into ionized fragments and detecting these fragments using their mass-to-charge ratio. A schematic diagram of Mass Spectrometry is shown in Figure 3.2.

These two components, used together, allow a much finer degree of substance identification than either unit used separately. It is not possible to make an accurate identification of a particular molecule by gas chromatography or mass spectrometry alone. The mass spectrometry process normally requires a very pure sample while gas chromatography using a traditional detector (e.g., FID) cannot differentiate between multiple molecules that happen to take the same amount of time to travel through the column (i.e., have the same retention time), which results in two or more molecules that co-elute. Sometimes two different molecules can also have a similar pattern of ionized fragments in a mass spectrometer (mass spectrum). Combining the two processes reduces the possibility of error, as it is extremely unlikely that two different molecules will behave in the same way in both a gas chromatograph and a mass spectrometer. Therefore, when an identifying mass spectrum appears at a characteristic retention time in a GC-MS analysis, it typically increases the certainty that the analyte of interest is in the sample. As a result, the GC-MS is a preferred technique over GC-FID in the analysis of isocyanates in a laboratory.

3.3.4. High-Performance Liquid Chromatography

High-performance liquid chromatography is a powerful technique capable of separating compounds that are not suitable for gas chromatography. The mixture containing analytes along with the mobile phase is pumped at high pressure through the separation column. The separation takes place in the column packed with tiny particles of porous silica. Different compounds move at different speeds through affinity to the two phases and then the compounds become separated. The different columns with different stationary phases are used to separate different types of compounds. From the column, the solvent and separated samples pass through the detector. HPLC as a separation technique is coupled to either a UV/ECD detector or a mass spectrometry for the detection of isocyanates derivatives.

In 2004, the field of separation science (High-Performance Liquid Chromatograph, HPLC) was revolutionised with the introduction of Ultra-performance Liquid Chromatograph [UPLC]. Significant advances in instrumentation and column technology were made to achieve dramatic increases in resolution, speed, and sensitivity in liquid chromatography. For the first time, a holistic approach involving simultaneous innovations in particle technology and instrument design was endeavoured to meet and overcome the challenges of the analytical laboratory. This was done to make analytical scientists more successful and businesses more profitable and productive. This new technology has been applied in the analysis of isocyanates using UPLC-MS/MS [Hu et al., 2014; Bhandari et al., 2016; Lepine et al., 2020]. A more detailed example will be provided in the later chapters.

3.3.5. Ultra-Violet/Electrochemical Detections

Many compounds such as isocyanate derivatives in solution absorb visible light and/or UV light. A UV detector coupled to an HPLC continuously measures the intensity of light with a specific wavelength passing through the mobile phase containing the isocyanate derivatives, and compares them to the intensity of the light before they were passed through the sample [HSE MDHS 25, 2014]. Since compounds will absorb specific wavelengths, they can be identified according to absorbance.

There are three different types of UV detectors: fixed wavelength detectors that rely on distinct wavelengths, and variable and photodiode array detectors that rely on one or more wavelengths generated from a broad spectrum lamp. Fixed wavelength detectors, the backbone of early HPLC systems, are cheap and simple, but are in limited use today. The most common fixed wavelength detectors use the 254 nm output from a low-pressure mercury lamp, the reason being many variable wavelength and photodiode array applications today still use this wavelength out of sheer habit. Photodiode array detectors (PDA) have an optical path similar to variable wavelength detectors except that the light passes through the flow cell prior to hitting the grating, allowing it to spread the spectrum across an array of photodiodes. Nowadays, UV detectors are most used and accepted as near 'universal' at low UV wavelengths. The applications of PDA peak purity can check the homogeneity of the samples. The features of spectral library searches, contour maps and 3D spectral display make the UV detectors easy to use. The cost of UV detectors is small, but it is very reliable. On the other hand, the compounds to be analysed by UV detectors must have a chromophore. Solvents used in mobile phases are required to be transparent. There are widely varying responses for different solutes.

Except for UV detectors, ECD is also widely used in the analysis of isocyanate derivatives. Target compounds (analytes) are separated using a separation column and mobile phase on an HPLC. After separation, the compounds present within the mobile phase enter the ECD. For compounds that can be oxidised or reduced the ECD is one of the most sensitive and selective HPLC detectors available. EC detectors require the use of electrically conductive HPLC mobile phases (buffers suffice) and, when properly used and maintained, are the standard bearer when it comes to response levels for the HPLC analysis of compounds such as catecholamines and neurotransmitters. EC detectors for HPLC usually contain three separate electrodes: a working, a counter (auxiliary), and a reference electrode. Common electrode materials are carbon, gold, silver, or platinum. A fixed potential difference is applied between the working electrode and the reference electrode to drive an electrochemical reaction at the working electrode's surface. Currently produced from the electrochemical reaction as compounds are oxidised or reduced at the working electrode is balanced by a current flowing in the opposite direction at the counter electrode. The EC detector response output is the amplified current resulting from the electrochemical reaction at the working electrode. The ECD detects this electrical current which linearly correlates to the analyte concentration loaded into the HPLC.

The advantages of ECD are that they are very sensitive and capable of detecting in the pg/L range depending on the analyte and sample matrix. By choosing the appropriate applied voltage for the oxidation/reduction potential and material of the working electrode, a more chemical-specific detecting condition can be obtained. At the same time, the mobile phase used in ECD analysis must be conductive, susceptible to background noise and electrode fouling. They are only applicable to compounds that can be oxidized or reduced.

3.3.6. Tandem Mass Spectrometer

Like GC-MS, when LC is combined with an MS detector, the tandem overcomes the LC with a lack of specification and delivers the advantage of identification. A highly sensitive concomitant detector with good specificity is the tandem mass spectrometer (LC-MS/MS).

Mass spectrometry is an analytical technique that measures the mass-to-charge ratio (m/z) of charged particles (ions). Although there are many kinds of mass spectrometers, all of them make use of electric or magnetic fields to manipulate the motion of ions produced from an analyte of interest and determine their m/z. The basic components of a mass spectrometer are the ion source, the mass analyser, the detector, and the data and vacuum systems. The ion source is where the components of a sample introduced in an MS system are ionized by means of electron beams, photon beams (UV lights), laser beams or corona discharge. In the case of electrospray ionization, the ion source moves ions that exist in liquid solution into the gas phase. The ion source converts and fragments the neutral sample molecules into gas-phase ions that are sent to the mass analyser. While the mass analyser applies the electric and magnetic fields to sort the ions by their masses, the detector measures and amplifies the ion current to calculate the abundance of each mass-resolved ion. In order to generate a mass spectrum that a human eye can easily recognize, the data system records, processes, stores, and displays data in a computer.

When the second phase of mass fragmentation is added, for example using the second quadrupole in a quadrupole instrument, it is called tandem MS (MS/MS). MS/MS can sometimes be used to quantitate low levels of target compounds in the presence of a high sample matrix background.

The first quadrupole (Q1) relates to a collision cell (Q2) and another quadrupole (Q3). Both quadrupoles can be used in scanning or static mode, depending on the type of MS/MS analysis being performed. Types of analysis include product ion scan, precursor ion scan, selected reaction monitoring (SRM) (sometimes referred to as multiple reaction monitoring (MRM)) and neutral loss scan. For example: When Q1 is in static mode (looking at one mass only as in SIM), and Q3 is in scanning mode, one obtains a so-called product ion spectrum (also called "daughter spectrum"). From this spectrum, one can select a prominent product ion which can be the product ion for the chosen precursor ion. The pair is called a 'transition' and forms the basis for SRM. SRM is highly specific and virtually eliminates matrix background. Figure 3.3 shows how a single quadrupole mass spectrometer (LC-MS) and a triple quadrupole mass spectrometer (LC-MS/MS) work, respectively

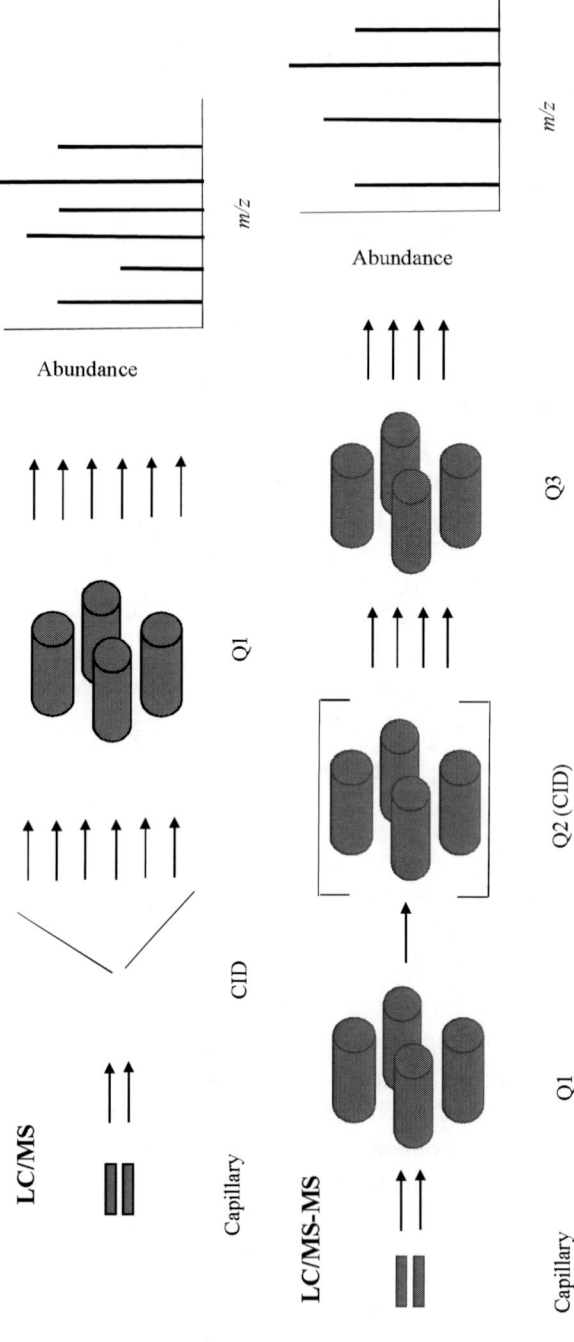

Figure 3.3. Comparison of single quadrupole mass spectrometer (LC-MS) and triple quadrupole mass spectrometer (LC-MS/MS).

The mass spectrum can be used to determine the mass of the analytes, their elemental and isotopic composition, or to elucidate the chemical structure of the sample. MS is an experiment that must take place in the gas phase and under a vacuum. Therefore, the development of devices facilitating the transition from samples at a higher pressure and in condensed phase (solid or liquid) into a vacuum system has been essential to developing MS as a potent tool for the identification and quantification of organic compounds and peptides. MS is now in very common use in analytical laboratories that study the physical, chemical, or biological properties of a wide variety of compounds. Among the many kinds of mass analysers, the ones that find application in LC-MS systems are the quadrupole, time-of-flight (TOF), ion traps, and hybrid quadrupole-TOF (QTOF) analysers.

Mass separation of the substances ionised by different interfaces has usually been performed using quadruple filters and quadrupole ion traps, and the use of other mass analysers such as time-of-flight (TOF) has recently started to increase. The full scan and high-resolution capabilities of QTOF instruments permit the possibility of developing non-target screening methods for biomarkers of exposure without any prior knowledge of the type of exposure suffered by individual. High-resolution full scan spectra data are acquired first, and later checked for the presence of any potential isocyanate metabolites generated after exposure, using their exact masses to enhance confidence in the result. In the case of a possible positive sample, using QTOF analysis, the product ion spectra in accurate mass are obtained to provide further evidence of the chemical structure of the metabolite. In addition, with the data acquired it would be feasible to identify unknown compounds in the samples investigated with the help of powerful software packages, although this subject is still a challenge for analytical chemists [Ibanez et al., 2005].

The interface between a HPLC with a continuously flowing elute, and a gas phase technique carried out in a vacuum was difficult for a long time. The advent of electrospray ionisation changed this. Currently, the most common LC-MS interfaces are ESI, APCI, and APPI. These are newer MS ion sources that facilitate the transition from a HPLC to high vacuum conditions needed at the MS analyser. In the ESI interface for LC-MS, it can be used for the analysis of moderately polar molecules (e.g., metabolites, xenobiotics, and peptides). The APCI ion source/interface can be used to analyse small, neutral, relatively non-polar, and thermally stable molecules (e.g., steroids, lipids, and fat-soluble vitamins). These compounds are not well ionised using ESI. APPI is another LC-MS ion source/interface for the analysis of neutral compounds that cannot be ionised using ESI. This interface is like the APCI ion source, but instead of a corona discharge, the ionisation occurs by using photons coming from a discharge lamp.

The coupling of MS with LC systems is attractive because liquid chromatography can separate delicate and complex natural mixtures, and chemical composition needs to be well established (e.g., biological fluids, environmental samples, and drugs).

3.4. Examples of Analytical Methods

Gas chromatograph or high-performance liquid chromatograph as a separation technique coupled to either UV/ECD detectors or a mass spectrometer is the preferred method for the detection of isocyanates from a range of different matrices. Examples of widely used analytical methods are described below.

3.4.1. Method for Assessing Airborne Isocyanates as -NCO Group by LC-UV-ECD

Immediately after sampling the filters are placed in vials containing 1,2-MP to completely cover the filter. This is done to ensure complete derivatisation of any residual free isocyanates. The sample filters are kept away from light and stored in a refrigerator until analysis.

The samples are analysed for total isocyanate content (expressed as -NCO group) at the laboratory. The procedure uses high-performance liquid chromatography, in accordance with the method described in MDHS 25/4 [HSE MDHS 25. 2014; Hu et al. 2014]. The detection limit for the method is established at 0.1 µg total-NCO in each filter sample. The method of sample preparation and the analytical procedure is briefly described below.

Sample preparation. Acetic anhydride of 100 µL is added into each glass vial containing the 1,2-MP desorbing solution and filter paper. The vial is mixed thoroughly and evaporated to dryness. The residue in a vial is dissolved in 2 mL acetonitrile or mobile phase. The solution is filtered into an HPLC sample vial using a 0.5 µm syringe filter.

Analytical procedure. An HPLC system with UV and EC detectors in series is used after sample extraction and concentration. The EC detector should be used in the oxidation mode. A diode array detector (DAD) is also recommended for confirmation and identification. Typical instrumental conditions and chromatograms (Figure 3.4) are given below.

Column	Kinetex C18, 5 µm, 4.6 x 250 mm
Mobile phase A	Sodium acetate buffer (60 Mm)
Mobile phase B	Acetonitrile
HPLC program	55% A and 45% B, Isocratic
Injection volume	20 µL
Column temperature	40°C
Flow rate	1 mL/min
UV detector	242 nm and/or DAD
EC detector	Graphite electrode, operating potential of + 0.8 V

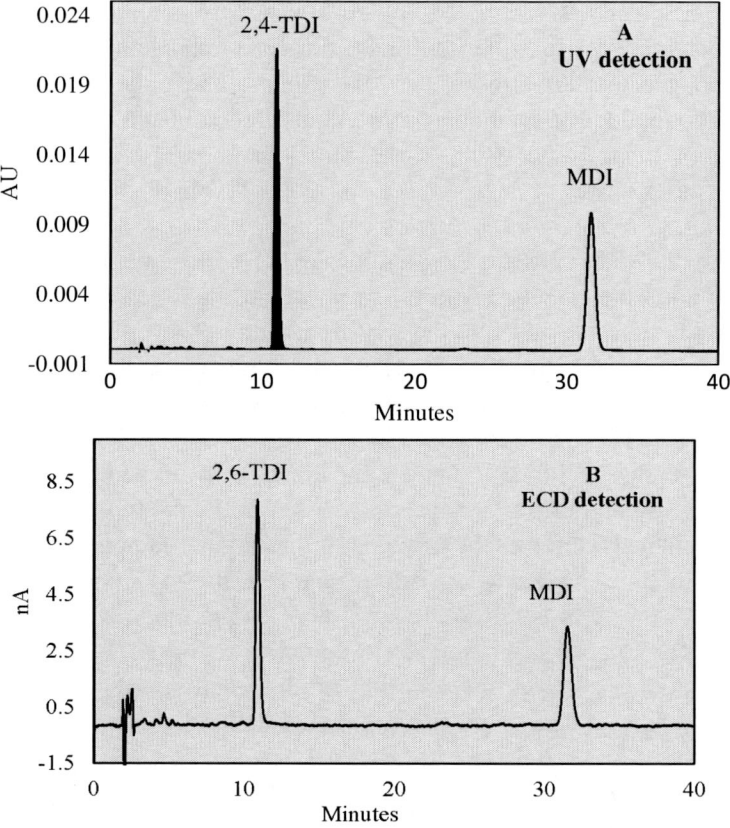

Figure 3.4. The chromatogram of LC-UV (A) LC-ECD and (B) of 2,6-TDI and MDI 1,2-MP derivatives [Hu et al., 2014].

Isocyanate-derivatised (1,2-MP) peaks can be identified based on the ratio EC and UV responses; by DAD spectral library matching and comparison with derivatised bulk formulations (where available). Quantification can be achieved by comparison with the relevant isocyanate monomer standard. Total isocyanate in air concentration is then determined from the sum of all the isocyanate-derived peaks.

3.4.2. Method for Assessing Airborne Both Isocyanate Monomers and Oligomers by LC-MS-MS

The procedure [Sigma-Aldrich Co. LLC. 2013] provides the steps for the extraction and analysis of the ASSET EZ4-NCO Dry sampler for isocyanates. The procedure describes the steps needed for the successful extraction of the DBA-isocyanate derivatives from the filters, preparation of calibration standards, and LC-MS method parameters. It is recommended that an adequate number of blank samplers from the same lot number be put through the workup and analysis.

Sample Preparation (Extraction Procedure). The red head-shrink tubing to access the filter cassette is carefully cut. The filter media from both the denuder and filter cassette is carefully removed using tweezers. The following reagent solutions are added to the centrifuge tubes. They are 3.0 mL of 1mM H_2SO_4, 3.0 mL of methanol, 5.5 mL of toluene (using the complete 5.5 mL to rinse the empty denuder into the centrifuge tubes), and 100 µL of 0.3 µg/mL deuterated ISTD. The tubes are shaken for 5 minutes, sonicated for 10 minutes, re-shaken for 20 minutes, and finally centrifuged for 10 minutes. After centrifuging, the top toluene layer is removed, and it is placed in a new tube. Another 5.5 mL toluene is added to the original sample. The operation steps of shaking, sonicating, re-shaking, and centrifuging are repeated. Again, the top toluene layer is removed, and it is placed in the previously collected toluene. The toluene is evaporated to complete dryness. The dry residue is reconstituted in 1.0 mL of acetonitrile and the resulting solution is sonicated for ~15 min and is then to be analysed by LC-MS/MS.

Analytical Procedure. A Sciex ExionLC system coupled with a Sciex Qtrap 5500 mass spectrometer is used for the analysis.

Typical operation conditions of LC and MS are given below:

LC conditions

Column	Ascentis Express C18, 2.7 µm, 2.1 x 50 mm			
Mobile phase A	5% ACN : 95% water with 0.05% formic acid			
Mobile phase B	95% ACN : 5% water with 0.05% formic acid			
Gradient	T (mins)	Flow Rate (mL/min)	A (%)	B (%)
	0	0.35	60	40
	2.0	0.35	20	80
	5.0	0.35	20	80
	5.1	0.35	0	100
	10.0	0.35	0	100
	10.1	0.35	60	40
	12.0	0.35	60	40
Injection volume	2 µL			
Column temperature	30°C			

MS conditions

Curtain Gas	30
Ion source	Electrospray Positive (ESI+)
Collision gas	medium
Ion Spray V	5500
Collision energy	Various for different ions
Entrance Energy (eV)	10
Desolvation temperature	450°C
Ion Source Gas 1	50 L/Hr
Ion Source Gas 2	60 L/Hr

Precursor ion, $[M + H]^+$	Product ions (m/z)	Collision energy (eV)	Declustering Potential, V	CXP
HDI 427.1	130.1	37	200	12
	156.2	31	200	13
2,6-TDI 434.4	130.1	29	180	12
	156.2	33	200	12
2,4-TDI 434.4	130.1	29	180	12
	156.2	33	200	12
MDI 509.4	130.1	35	250	13
	156.2	26	250	13
HDI Uretidone 724.6	130.2	40	150	15
	156.2	46	200	14
HDI Isocyanurate 892.6	130.2	44	200	12
	156.2	52	200	12
MDI 3 ring 769.7	130.2	31	230	15
	156.2	40	230	15
MDI 4 ring 1030.0	130.2	42	160	13
	156.2	54	160	13

Another example of the application of LC-MS/MS used in the analysis of isocyanates by air monitoring is shown in Figure 3.5.

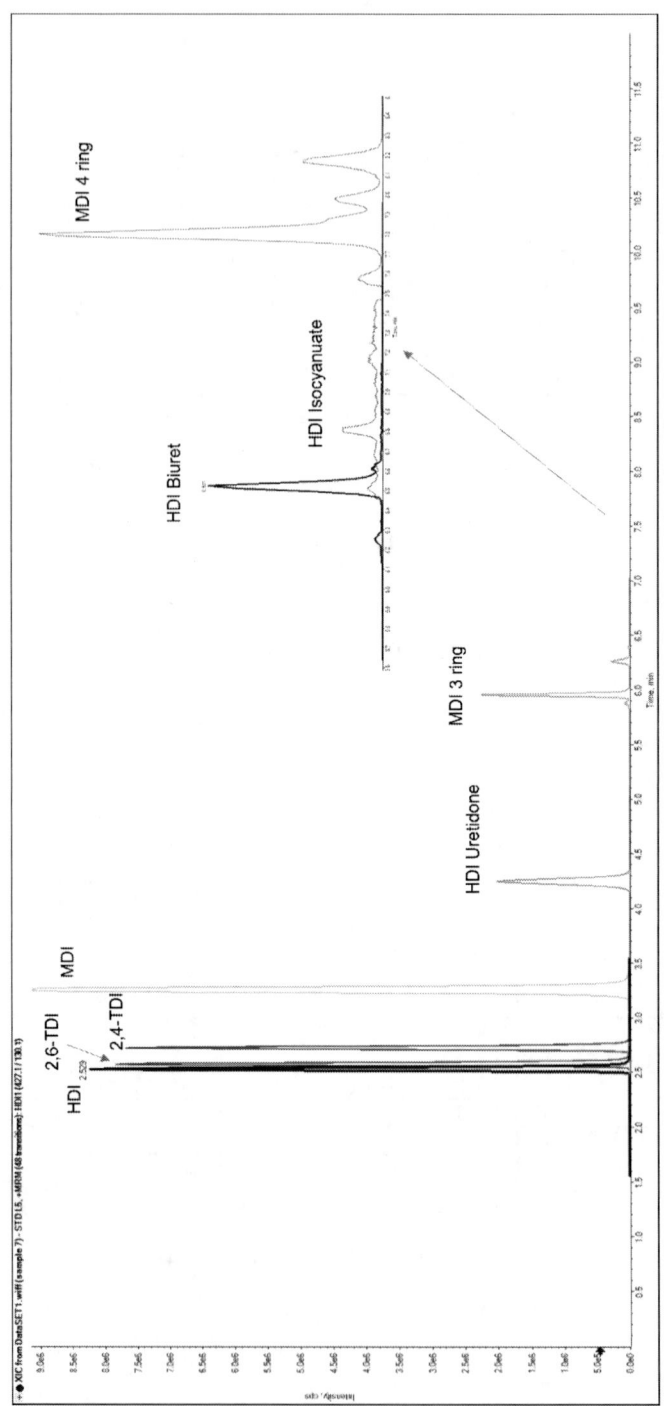

Figure 3.5. The application of LC-MS/MS is used in the analysis of isocyanates by air monitoring.

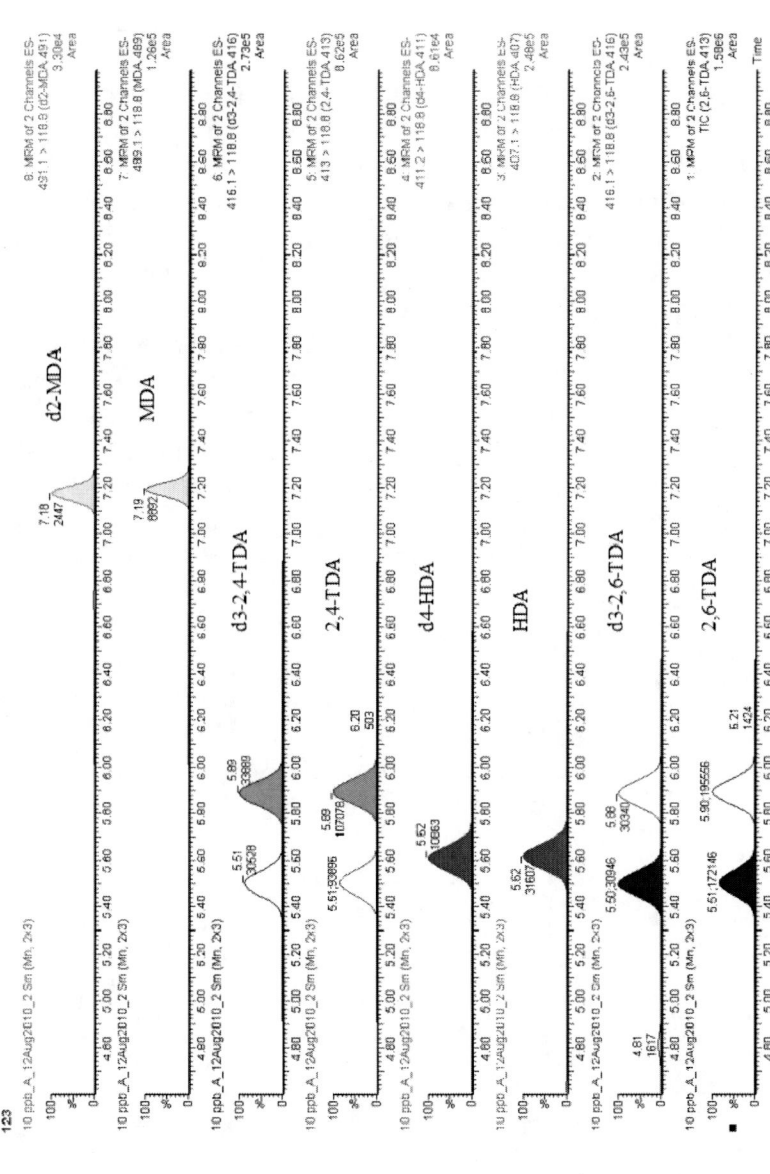

Figure 3.6. LC-MS/MS chromatograms of work-up urine samples spiked with amines at 10 µg/L and with the deuterium-labelled amines at 5 µg/L [Hu et al., 2014].

3.4.3. Method for Assessing Biomarkers of Exposure to Isocyanates by LC-MS/MS

Urine samples are collected at the end of the work shift. The samples are kept away from light and stored in a freezer until analysis.

A highly sensitive and specific ultra-high performance liquid chromatograph-tandem mass spectrometry method is used for the determination of the isocyanate-derived amines in urine samples [Hu 2014]. The method has a low limit of quantitation of 0.5 µg isocyanate-derived diamine/L. The method of sample preparation and analytical procedure is briefly described below.

Sample preparation. The work-up procedure of the urine samples was performed using a modified version of the protocol developed [Marand et al., 2004; Williams et al., 1999; Hu et al., 2014]. Briefly, an aliquot of a urine sample is hydrolysed by heating to 100°C for 2.5 hours. Prior to the hydrolysis, an aliquot of internal standards containing each of the deuterium-labelled amines is added to the urine solution. After hydrolysis, the samples are extracted into toluene by the addition of saturated NaOH solution. The samples are shaken and centrifuged. The organic layer is transferred to new test tubes, perfluoro fatty acid anhydride is added and the mixture is immediately shaken. The excess of the reagent and the acid formed are removed by extraction with a phosphate buffer solution. The organic phase, containing the amide derivatives, is evaporated to dryness. The dry residue is reconstituted into acetonitrile. The sample solutions are subsequently transferred to vials and analysed using UPLC-MS/MS.

Analytical Procedure. A Waters ACQUITY UPLC system with a Quattro Premier XE triple quadrupole mass spectrometer was used for the analysis.

Typical operation conditions of LC and MS are given below:

LC conditions

Column	UPLC BEH C18, 1.7 µm, 2.1 x 150 mm			
Mobile phase A	5% ACN : 95% Water			
Mobile phase B	5% Water : 95% ACN			
Gradient	T (mins)	Flow Rate (mL/min)	A (%)	B (%)
	0	0.35	70	30
	0.5	0.35	70	30
	5.0	0.35	30	70
	8.5	0.35	30	70
	8.6	0.35	70	30
	10.0	0.35	70	30

Injection volume	10 µL partial loop over-fill, Air gap: 1.0 µL of pre-aspirate and 0.0 µl of post-aspirate, Needle overfill flush: 3.0 µL.
Weak wash	Mobile phase A
Strong wash	90% Methanol: 10% Water
Column temp	40°C

MS conditions

Capillary	3.0 kV
Ion source	Electrospray Negative (ESI-)
Source temperature	120°C
Collision gas pressure	3.5 e^{-3} mbar
Collision energy	Various for different ions
Desolvation temperature	350°C
Cone gas flow	50 L/Hr
Desolvation gas flow	700 L/Hr
Dwell time	0.01 or 0.02 s

Precursor ion, [M - H]-	Product ions (m/z)	Cone voltage (V)	Collision energy (eV)
2,6 TDA 413	118.8	30	30
	293	30	20
HDA 407.1	118.8	30	25
	287.1	30	15
2,4 TDA 413	118.8	30	30
	293	30	20
MDA 489.1	118.8	30	30
	369.1	30	20

The typical LC-MS/MS chromatograms of urine samples spiked with amines at 10 µg/L and with the deuterium-labelled amines at 5 µg/L are demonstrated in Figure 3.6.

MassLynx (Waters) software with automated processing (QuanLynx) was used running in the MRM mode. The analytes were identified by two characteristic MRM transitions: their ion ratio and retention time. Tolerance was set to ± 20% for the ion ratio and ± 1% for the retention time. Quantification was performed by integration of the area under the curve from the specific MRM chromatograms of the analytes and their internal standard. The response (the ratio of the integrated area of the analyte and the corresponding IS) was compared to the calibration curve.

There is another example of analysis of isocyanate metabolites (HDA) in urine using GC/MS technique [Williams et al., 1999]. The analytical method is described briefly below. An exposed urine sample was hydrolysed with acid first and then cooled, followed by adding NaOH. After hydrolysis, diethyl ether was added and the samples were extracted. The organic layer was transferred and evaporated. Samples were then resuspended in toluene and derivatised with heptafluorobutyric anhydride. Samples were cooled, evaporated to dryness, and reconstituted in toluene. The samples were analysed by GC-MS with negative ion chemical ionisation. Samples were injected onto a BP-5 fused silica capillary column. The oven temperature ramped from 150°C to 280°C at 10°C/min where it was held for 1.5 minutes. The interface temperature was 180°C and the source was held at 200°C. With selected ion monitoring, ion m/z 449 was monitored for HAD and m/z 462 for HpDA (internal standard). This method gave a detection limit of 1 μg/L.

3.5. Laboratory Accreditation and Quality Control/Assurance

Since 1972 American Industrial Hygiene Association (AIHA) has had a laboratory accreditation program. To be accredited, a laboratory must implement and maintain a quality management system that complies with ISO/IEC 17025 (2017) and AIHA modules applicable to the laboratory's scope of analysis. The system typically will be described in a quality manual and associated policies and procedures. These documents must address 8 management system requirements such as management system documentation, control of management system documents, control of records, actions to address risks and opportunities, improvement, corrective actions, internal audits, and management reviews. In addition, there are several technical requirements addressing method selection and validation, equipment calibration, routine quality control (QC), determination of method uncertainty, traceability of measurements, reporting of results, etc. The QC program requires records demonstrating regular analysis of QC samples and statistical treatment of QC data. Laboratory compliance with these requirements is verified during biannual on-site assessments of each laboratory. Participation in and maintenance of proficiency in the appropriate proficiency testing programs is also required.

Attaining reliable results from air and biological samples is not an easy task. The low analyte levels often require complex treatment procedures that must be carried out with a high degree of precision to allow reliable assessment of exposure. An approach widely applied today to achieve, maintain, and document the quality of work of an analytical laboratory is the adoption of a quality control program [ISO17025]. Internal quality control and external quality assurance are important parts of quality management.

1. One of the most popular external quality assurance systems for chemical substances and their metabolites is run by the Institute and Outpatient Clinic for Occupational, Social and Environmental Medicine of the University of Erlangen-Nuremberg, Germany, G-EQUAS. This scheme comprises the determination of HDA, 2,4-TDA, 2,6-TDA and MDA in urine samples. A laboratory takes part in the program twice a year. About 200 laboratories from more than 35 countries regularly participate in this scheme.
2. In addition, RECIPE Chemicals & Instruments GmbH in Germany provides the ClinChek Controls which are intended to ensure the accuracy and precision of daily laboratory results. Unlike the G-EQUAS scheme which has 4 diamines of isocyanate metabolites, the Controls consist of only MDA.
3. Institut de recherche Robert-Sauve en sante et en sacurite du travail (Occupational Health and Safety Research Institute), Canada. The programs are mainly for workplace samples.

A key component of the laboratory accreditation program is required for laboratories to participate in appropriate proficiency testing (PT) programs to demonstrate their ability to provide acceptable results. The Proficiency Analytical Testing (PAT) program provides PT samples for various chemical tests.

3.6. Discussion

3.6.1. Ultra/Violet and Electrochemical Detections Verse Mass Spectrometer

One of the most widely used methods for determining isocyanates in air is the MDHS 25 method [HSE MDHS 25, 2014; White, 2006b]. The method is the quantification of isocyanates (NCO) as their 1-(2-methoxyphenyl) piperazine (1,2-MP) derivatives. Monomeric NCO-MP, for which a suitable standard exists or can be prepared is measured by UV or EC detection in series. UV detection is simpler to use and gives a less variable response than EC detection but is less sensible. In the method, monomeric and oligomeric NCO-MP derivatives are quantified by the EC detector using the response factor obtained from the relevant MP-derivertised monomer. However, most laboratories across the world use UV detection for the quantification of NCO-

MP derivatives as UV detectors are widespread and relatively easy to use [Hu et al., 2014].

For the purpose of confirmation, peaks are identified as being derivatised isocyanates by using the ratio of the response of EC and UVdetectors for the derivatised polymer and monomer and comparing this ratio with an empirically derived range. The use of this EC/UV ratio approach preexists with the widespread availability of liquid chromatography/mass spectrometry (LC/MS). The validity of the EC/UV ratio is regarded as a "poor man's MS" [White, 2006a].

When UPLC technology is used in the analysis of biomarkers to exposure of isocyanates [Hu et al., 2014], the analytical column used in the method had a very small particle size (< 2 μm) giving narrow chromatographic peaks with an average peak width of 0.2 min (Figure 3.6). This gave higher sensitivity and good separation of the four isocyanate-derivatised amines in a relatively short time (8 minutes) comparing the previous method [Marand et al., 2004] in which a conventional column was used with a 30 minute run.

Mass spectrometry is a detection technique that is based on the measurement of the mass-to-charge (m/z) ratio of ionised analyte molecules. The obtained m/z ratio from analytes can then be identified by correlating the mass with that of a specific molecule and/or by identifying characteristic fragmentation patterns that may occur during ionisation. LC-MS/MS has the advantage in combination with high sensitivity and high selectivity. This is essential for the analysis of low-concentration analytes in a complex matrix such as urine. With matrices that have a lower expectation of interfering compounds, such as air samples, some studies use LC-UV/EC detectors. The selectivity of UV/ECD for isocyanates is described as feasible for air samples [HSE MDHS 25. 2014]. Although, ECD can be at least 100 times more sensitive towards responsive compounds than a standard UV detector and much more selective, with time electrochemical reaction products tend to accumulate at the electrode surface leading to loss of activity and hence a loss of detector response. This is the major reason why UV and EC detectors are combined for the analysis of airborne isocyanates samples, in which UV is used for confirmation and ECD for quantitation. However, this combination detection method generally suffers from a slightly lower limit of detection than MS, and a lower selectivity, especially in complex matrices (Table 3.1).

Laboratory Analytical Methods 51

Table 3.1. Detection sensitivity comparison between two Methods for Determining Isocyanate Concentrations in Air

	Asset EZ4-NCO	HSE MDHS 25/3
Analysis Detection	HPLC with MS/MS	HPLC with UVD/ECD
Quantitation Limit	0.03 ng TDIs/ml, 0.5 ng HDI/ml, 2.0 ng MDI/ml	10 ng HDI, TDIs and MDI per sample
Limit of Detection	0.002 µg TDIs/m3, 0.03 µg HDI/m^3, 0.1 µg MDI/m^3 (15 L)	1 µg HDI, TDIs and MDI/m^3, (15 L)

A highly sensitive mass detector with good specificity is the LC/MS/MS but the cost is prohibitive. HPLC-ECD has the perfect balance of price and performance for routine measurements of workplace samples in the determination of airborne isocyanates.

3.6.2. Gas Chromatograph-Mass Spectrometer verse Liquid Chromatograph-Mass Spectrometer

Isocyanate metabolites (amines) are non-volatile, polar compounds that are not suitable for application of GC-MS. This has been overcome by using derivatisation of amines during the sample preparation. For a quite long time, GC-MS has been the "golden-standard" for detection [Cocker et al., 2017]

Isocyanate metabolites (amines) are non-volatile, polar compounds, characteristics that make liquid chromatography/mass spectrometry (LC-MS) the technique of choice [Marand et al., 2004; Hu et al., 2014, 2017; Bhandari et al., 2016; Lepine et al., 2020].

When analysing derivatised isocyanates by LC coupled to tandem MS, a majority of the applications use an ESI as an ionisation source [Marand et al., 2004; Hu et al., 2014]. ESI as an ionisation technique has the advantage of very little in-source fragmentation. It means that the molecular ion can always be observed. When combining the ESI with MS/MS, the possibility to quantify analytes collision-induced disassociation methods can be used to further enhance selectivity. This selected reaction mode (SRM), which is also known as multiple reaction monitoring (MRM) depends on the instrument vendor, requires a selected intact analyte molecular ion after the ionisation to pass through the first analyser, in order to be fragmented in a collision cell to allow the second analyser to detect its specific product ions.

There are a number of benefits for the use of LC-MS for quantification. First, combining the two separation mechanisms of LC and MS allows for the analysis of complex mixtures. The resulting selectivity allows particular analytes or analytes to be isolated from the mixture and gives confidence that the correct component is being measured. Since analytes are separated by their mass-to-charge (m/z) the technique allows for the use of isotopically labelled internal standards, which may not be separated by LC but can be separated by their mass difference. The use of stable isotopically labelled internal standards can help control variability in a quantitative assay. Second, since the MS will distinguish compounds based on mass, the chromatographic method does not have to separate every single component in the sample, so co-elution of non-isobaric analytes is possible. This allows fast LC analysis times and reduced sample preparation, which helps with method development and high throughput sample analysis. Third, mass spectrometry is an inherently sensitive technique. Good selectivity also leads to reduced noise, allowing very low levels (pg/L) to be detected.

On the other hand, there are disadvantages to the use of LC-MS. First, mass spectrometers that can couple to LC systems are expensive to buy and run. Regular servicing is also required, adding to the cost. The environmental conditions in the laboratory need to be well controlled to ensure system stability. Second, in their own right, both LC and MS can be difficult to optimise. Combining the two leads to a complex co-dependant synergy. The ionisation mechanism can be especially complicated – often several species are formed in the ionisation source and multiple charging can occur. Care must be taken to choose conditions for optimum sensitivity and reproducibility. Sufficient training is also needed to allow analysts to run the systems effectively. Third, compared to the other quantitative techniques LC-MS can give a limited range where the response is linear with respect to concentration. Typically, ranges should not exceed 500-fold concentrations. Last, in quantitative analysis, it is usual that the MS is set to only detect specific analytes. This results in a very "clean" looking chromatogram and it is easy to forget that there can be a lot of components still present, but not seen. These components can cause problems with reproducible quantitation and can be difficult to trace if they are not being looked for.

As the examples of applications of both GC-MS and LC-MS in the analysis of isocyanates in air monitoring and biological monitoring demonstrate, it is worthwhile discussing the differences between these two types of techniques.

GC and LC are both chromatography separation techniques that are immensely popular with the analytical chemist. Over the last several decades, mass spectroscopy has contributed significantly to the scope of applications of both GC and LC. Hyphenated mass spectroscopy techniques have made possible separation and identification of complex mixtures in a matter of minutes, which in earlier days would take several hours, if not days.

GC-MS has proven to be a valuable tool for the analysts of volatile compounds which are stable enough to withstand high temperatures during gas chromatographic separations. On the other hand, LC-MS is suitable for compounds of lower volatility whose volatility cannot be increased even on derivatisation. Both GC-MS and LC-MS are advanced chromatographic techniques that are used for the separation of complex sample mixtures. After ionisation, the ionised fragments are led through mass filters to the detector.

The number of dissimilarities is more and need a clear understanding to help laboratory chemists take a judicious choice in the separation of the technique to meet their analysis requirements. The differences between of two techniques are discussed briefly below.

- *Mobile phase*. It is obvious that GC-MS makes use of an inert gas as a carrier whereas LC-MS uses a mixture of liquids with or without buffers or additives as a carrier phase.
- *Nature of compounds*. GC-MS is suitable for the analysis of samples of essential oils, fatty acids, alcohols, polysaccharides, esters, terpenes, flavours and gases. LC-MS has no known applications for the analysis of gases but common applications include nonpolar compounds such as amines, nucleotides, nucleosides, steroids and other molecules of biological interest.
- *Vacuum requirements*. Vacuum requirements are more stringent for LC-MS as any liquid in the carrier stream needs to be removed totally before sample constituents are allowed to proceed to the ionization chamber. This requires fine control of the vacuum through multiple pumps in LC-MS. In the case of GC-MS as the carrier is a gas, such high vacuum requirements are not necessary.
- *Ionisation techniques*. Electron impact is the common ionization mode in GC-MS and chemical ionisation is also available as a soft ionization option. Electrospray ionization and atmospheric pressure chemical ionization are preferred ionization techniques in LC-MS systems.

- *Spectral libraries.* The spectral match is facilitated through the availability of libraries on classes of compounds for the positive identification of components. Such databases are commonly available from global standard bodies such as NIST. However, such libraries are rarely available for LC-MS systems but one can create their own spectral search libraries depending on the analytical requirements. Typical analyses such as forensic applications require confirmation on the presence or absence of specific substances instead of complete sample composition so GC-MS is preferred because of its lower cost, ease of operation and maintenance. However, for demanding applications requiring identification and quantification at low concentrations of known and unknown components, LC-MS is the preferred choice.
- *Cost.* LC-MS systems are more expensive in comparison to G-MS. They require specialized operator training as well as more maintenance. On the other hand, G-MS is simpler to operate and requires less maintenance, as only components like septa and liners need replacement from time to time to maintain optimum performance.

The two methods [Willams et al., 1999 and Marand et al., 2004] are quite similar in the sample preparation phase which involves hydrolysis, extraction, derivatisation, evaporation, and reconstitution. However, the two techniques perform differently in the terms of the detection limit. The GC-MS gave 5 nmol/L but LC-MS/MS delivered 5×10^{-3} nmol/L. The sensitive determination in urine by LC-MS/MS is mainly due to the selective MS/MS-determination which reduces the matrix effects.

3.7. Conclusion

The next 5–10 years will inevitably witness increased inter-laboratory cooperation to collate as much LC-MS-based metabolite data as possible. In-house MS/MS libraries will likely become more available to interested collaborators with similar model samples and instrumentation, increasing the knowledge base of all participating laboratories. The integration of NMR to LC-MS-based metabolic profiling and metabolomic studies will likely increase, either through the offline analysis of collected LC fractions or through hybrid LCNMR-MS instrumentation. In contrast, GC-MS is unlikely to become an integrated component of an LC-MS strategy, due to the fundamental differences between the two techniques and the inherent difficulty in utilizing such complementary information for unknown biomarker characterization. However, GC-MS will remain a tool for quantifying those metabolites not amenable to LC-MS analysis due to relatively poor ionization efficiencies. New informatics tools for the combined automated generation of candidate empirical formula and stereoisomer generation for detected metabolite features may become available, as well as algorithms designed to predict the chemical structure of unknown metabolites based on CID MS/MS fragmentation spectra. However, the functional complexity of the metabolome has so far precluded the development of the latter.

Separately, QTOF mass analysers are seldom used in isocyanates analysis despite their improved resolution and mass accuracy characteristics, which make them very suitable for confirmation purposes. The main reasons for the relative unpopularity of QTOF MS in this field are its limited sensitivity and its high acquisition cost.

Chapter 4

Airborne Monitoring and Its Applications

4.1. Introduction

Isocyanates are extensively used in the automotive industry and in the manufacture and application of polyurethane. The most used isocyanate includes diisocyanates, and its oligomers are hexamethylene diisocyanate (HDI), toluene diisocyanate (TDI) and methylene diphenyl diisocyanate (MDI). HDI is used in two-pack spray paints while TDI and MDI are used in the manufacture of polyurethane foams, floor coverings and adhesives. In a large proportion of product formulations many diisocyanate monomers have been replaced by their oligomers, which have lower vapour pressure to reduce inhalation exposure [Pronk et al., 2006a and 2006b; Hu et al., 2017].

It is well known that these chemicals can cause respiratory sensitisation and asthma [McDonald et al., 2005; Dao and Benstein, 2018] and 3% of all Australian workers are likely exposed to isocyanates at work in their current job [El-Zaemey et al., 2018]. Efforts to reduce the incidence of isocyanate-induced asthma should focus on ensuring effective control measures in workplaces where isocyanates are being used. One of the ways to ensure effective control measures is to conduct the sampling and analysis of airborne isocyanates in workplaces. However, airborne isocyanate exposure assessment is a difficult task that poses some challenges for occupational hygiene professionals including the analytical chemists in the laboratory.

Exposure to isocyanates, leading to an increased risk of occupational asthma, has been a pertinent issue since its acknowledgement in the 1950s [Bernstein, 1982]. As such, sensitive and selective sampling and analysis of the isocyanate sensitising agent as well as monitoring at very low concentrations and short exposures has been in high demand due to the long withstanding awareness of isocyanate exposure risk.

Isocyanate sampling and analysis is challenging as its chemical and physical properties that exist as a vapour or aerosol constitute a wide range of particles and chemical species, such as monomers, dimers, oligomers, or the polymeric form. For airborne sampling of isocyanates, the first-generation method is an impinger method that is commonly recommended. This method uses a solvent medium to trap, dissolve, and derivative the isocyanate aerosols to help prevent an underestimation of isocyanates. Impinger methods are also recommended for processes that generate particles greater than 2 µm. However, the use of an impinger is inconvenient and are inherently hazardous, potentially exposing workers to solvents such as toluene and dimethyl sulfoxide. Furthermore, impinger solvents are potentially flammable. As a result, the impregnated filter method has been developed. The personal isocyanate samples are usually collected on filters by drawing a known volume of air through a glass fibre filter coated with a derivatising agent.

Over the last four decades, the National Institute for Occupational Safety and Health (NIOSH) or the Occupational Safety and Health Administration (OSHA) in the US, and the Health and Safety Executive (HSE) in the UK have been developing many sampling and analytical methods for airborne monitoring exposure to isocyanates to be suitable in various workplace conditions. In the last two decades, two commercial samplers have been developed (ISO-Chek and Asset EZ4-NCO). These samplers along with the impinger sampler are demonstrated in Figure 4.1.

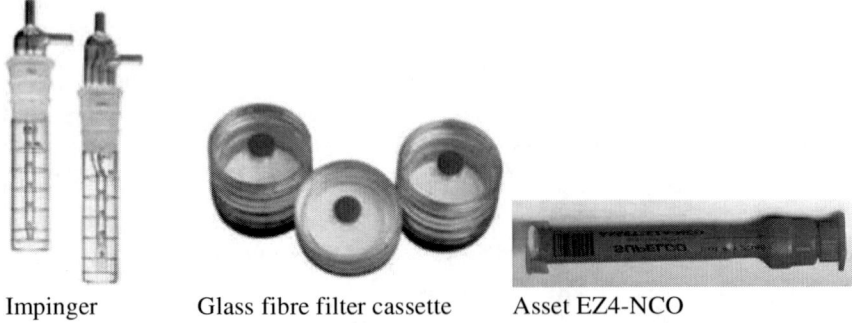

Impinger   Glass fibre filter cassette   Asset EZ4-NCO

Figure 4.1. Common sampling methods for isocyanates.

Recently, a new approach using CIP10M was developed [Puscasu et al., 2015a], therefore demonstrating the vast efforts in recent years to develop new sampling devices, novel derivatizing reagents, and analytical methods with lower detection.

Although several review papers have been published on selecting isocyanate sampling and analytical methods [Streicher et al., 1994 and 2002; Levine et al., 1995; Guglya 2000; Henneken et al., 2007, Bengtstrom et al., 2016], the most recent developments in the field – especially among the applications of three commonly used methods, Asset EZ4-NCO, HSE MDHS 25 and Iso-Chek have not yet been compared and summarised; these are covered in detail in this chapter. The future research goals in airborne isocyanate exposure monitoring are also discussed below.

4.2. Sampling and Analytical Methods

4.2.1. OSHA and NIOSH Methods

Since the 1980's, the OSHA and NIOSH in the USA and HSE in the UK have developed various samples and analytical methods to suit a variety of workplace environments (Table 4.1).

Table 4.1. Comparison of NIOSH and OSHA Isocyanate Methods

	NIOSH 2523	NIOSH 5521	NIOSH 5522	NIOSH 5525	OSHA42/47	OSHA 5002
Developed in	1987	1989	1996	2003	1983/1984	2020
Monomers Oligomers	TDI, HDI None	TDI, MDI, HDI, NDI, HMDI HDI	TDI, MDI, HDI, NDI, HMDI, IPDI TDI, MDI, HDI	NCO	42, TDI, HDI 47, MDI None	TDI, MDI, HDI, NDI, HMDI, IPDI TDI, MDI, HDI
Sampler	Coated glass wool/opaque tube	Impinger	Impinger	Coated GFF Impinger	Coated GFF	Coated GFF
Reagent Shelf Life	Nitro reagent 7d 25 C in dark	1,2-MP in toluene 7d 0 C	Tryptamine in DMSO 6 mo 25 C in dark	MAP in butyl benzoate 3 mo at -10 C in dark	1,2-PP 6 mo 0 C sealed	1,2-PP 2-8 C
Technique	HPLC UV	HPLC PDA/EC	HPLC FLR/EC	HPLC	HPLC FLR/UV	HPLC FLR

The NIOSH Method 2535 was first published in 1987 and uses p-nitrobenzyl-N-propylamine (nitro reagent) deposited on glass wool and packed in a sampling tube. The method is good mainly for monomeric aromatic isocyanate vapours but not aerosols [NIOSH 1987]. The NIOSH Method 5521 developed in 1989 consists of sampling into an impinger solution containing 1-(2-methoxyphenyl)-piperazine (1,2-MP) in toluene and determines the air concentration of specific isocyanates [NIOSH 1989]. The NIOSH Method 5522 published in 1996 consists of sampling into an impinger solution containing tryptamine in DMSO. The method determines the air concentration of monomers and estimates the concentration of oligomers of specific diisocyanates. It is applicable to vapours and aerosols. However, the solvent DMSO is readily absorbed into the skin making it unsafe for a worker to wear. Therefore, this method is designed for area sampling only and is not suitable for personal exposure sampling [NIOSH 1996]. This relatively new developed NIOSH Method 5525 in 2003 determines the air concentration of monomeric and oligomeric isocyanates which is similar in principle to other NIOSH methods. However, it differs from them in two aspects, whereby the reagent 1-(9-anthracenylmethyl)piperazine (MAP) and fluorescence detector (FLD) were used [NIOSH 2003, Bello et al., 2002]. The OSHA Method 42 was developed in 1983 for the determination of HDI, 2,4-TDI and 2,6-TDI [OSHA, 1983]. In the following year, MDI was developed in OSHA Method 47 [OSHA, 1984]. These two methods consist of sampling onto a glass fibre filter coated with 1-(2-pyridyl)-piperazine (1-2PP) which is contained in open-face cassettes. Samples are extracted with 90/10 (v/v) acetonitrile/dimethyl sulfoxide and analysed by high-performance liquid chromatography (HPLC) using an ultraviolet or fluorescence detector (UV or FLD). Most recently in 2020, the OSHA published a comprehensive method [OSHA 2022] covering OSHA 42/47 and adding up isocyanates oligomers analysis.

Apart from the above methods developed by OSHA and NIOSH in the US, three methods have been developed which are most widely used methods across the world in recent years. They are named HSE MDHS 25, Asset EZ4-NCO, and ISO-Chek. These methods include a variety of cassettes with impingers, treated filters, and denuders as summarised in Table 4.2.

4.2.2. Other Widely Used Methods

4.2.2.1. HSE MDHS 25 Method

The HSE has been involved in developing analytical methods for airborne isocyanates for over 30 years. The current UK method for isocyanate determination is the HSE method (Table 4.2), Methods for the Determination of Hazardous Substances, Organic Isocyanates in Air, HSE MDHS 25/4 [HSE MDHS 25, 2014]. Unlike the NIOSH and OSHA methods having multiple methods for different workplace circumstances, the HSE method uses one method to cover most of the workplace environment for the determination of isocyanates. The method that is probably the most used worldwide for the determination of organic NCO in the air is the HSE method [White et al., 2012]. This method traps the isocyanate with a 1,2-MP reagent to form the stable urea derivative by drawing workplace air through an impinger containing 1,2-MP solution and/or through an 1,2-MP impregnated filter. The procedure can be used for the determination of time-weighted average concentrations of organic isocyanates in workplace atmospheres. It is suitable for a wide range of organic compounds containing isocyanate functional groups. The principle of operation is described below. (1) A measured volume of air is drawn through a glass impinger containing 1,2-MP absorbing solution backed with a filter impregnated with 1,2-MP reagent (isocyanate aerosols) or alternatively a single filter impregnated with the 1,2-MP reagent (isocyanate vapour). The isocyanates present in the air will react with 1,2-MP to form non-volatile urea derivatives. (2) After extraction and concentration, the sample solutions can be analysed by HPLC with UV and electrochemical (EC) detection. Isocyanate-derived peaks can be identified based on the ratio of EC and UV responses; by diode array detection (DAD) spectral library matching and comparison with derivatised bulk formulations. (3) Quantification can be achieved by comparing with the relevant isocyanate monomer standard. Total isocyanate-in-air concentrations are then determined from the sum of all the isocyanate-derived peaks.

However, doubt has been raised about the capability of the HSE 25/3 method in peaks identified as being derivatised isocyanates by using the ratio of the response of UV and EC detectors for the derivatised polymer and monomers and comparing this ratio with an empirically derived range [Walker, 2007]. Moreover, ECD occasionally leads to issues with interferences whilst aerosols (impinger) are considered unsafe for personal

Table 4.2. Widely Used Methods for Determining Isocyanate Concentrations in Air.

	Asset EZ4-NCO	Iso-Chek	HSE MDHS 25/3
Sampler	13 mm filter + denuder	25 mm closed-face double filter cassette	25 mm Filter, impinger, or impinger+filter
Sample Media	GFF+Denuder/DBA	PTFE Filter traps aerosol phase, field derivatised with 1,2-MP, GFF impregnated with MAMA collects vapour phase	GFF/1,2-MP
Shelf life	Two years	10 months at ambient temperature	3 months
Flow Rate Sampling time	0.2 L/min (typical) (0.02 L/min – 0.85 mL/min) 15 minutes (typical) (5 minutes – 12 hours)	1 L/min 15 minutes	Impinger 1 L/min 15 min – 8 hours Filter 2 L/min 20 min – 15 hours
Analysis Detection	HPLC with MS or MS/MS	HPLC with FLD	HPLC with UVD/ECD
Limit of Detection (LOD)	0.002 µg TDIs/m3, 0.03 µg HDI/m^3, 0.1 µg MDI/m^3 (15 L)	0.01 µg/m^3 for TDIs, HDI, MDI monomers 0.1 µg/m^3 for HDI and MDI oligomers (15 L)	1 µg HDI, TDIs and MDI/m^3, (15 L)
Limit of Quantitation (LOQ)	0.03 ng TDIs/ml, 0.5 ng HDI/ml, 2.0 ng MDI/ml	0.15 ng/ml for TDIs, HDI, MDI, monomers 1.5 ng/ml for HDI and MDI oligomers	10 ng HDI, TDIs and MDI per sample
ISO	ISO 17734-1:2013	ISO 17736:2010	ISO16702-2:2012
Advantages	Easy to use and safe to wear, provide high capacity, suitable for sampling from 5 minutes to 8 hours, stable with two-year shelf life before sampling, no rush to the laboratory, stable after sampling for 4 weeks, samples both monomers and oligomers, achieve sensitivity and limits of detection 50 -100 times below existing methods	Ease of use, reduction of toluene risk from impinger collection methods and straightforwardness of lab analysis, ability to collect isocyanate monomers and oligomers, ability to collect particles and vapours	Widely recognised method, trapping the NCO with a derivatisation reagent, 1,2-MP, rapidly forms a stable urea and stable at room temperature, sampling vapour (filters) and sampling times long (8 hours) for TWA
Disadvantages	Sample preparation is quite involved, targeted analysis rather than total isocyanates	Short sampling time and needs field derivatisation	Aerosols (impinger) considered unsafe for personal sampling, 1,2-MP is a banned substance in the UK, interference on ECD

sampling and 1,2-MP is a banned substance in the UK. The recent development [HSE MDHS 25, 2014; White et al., 2012] shows that the liquid chromatography/tandem mass spectrometry (LC-MS/MS) offers significant advantages over the UV/EC version of MDHS 25/3 in that it is more sensitive, provides improved identification, and has been found to be easier to use.

Two commercial sampling methods and analytical methods have been developed and have become available in the last two decades (Table 4.2).

4.2.2.2. Iso-Chek Method

The Iso-Chek Isocyanate sampling systems developed by SKC Inc was the first commercially available sampler that could determine isocyanates in air. It is a preloaded three-piece cassette that contains two stages. Stage one contains an untreated polytetrafluoroethylene (PTFE) filter to collect the aerosol phase, and stage two holds a glass fibre filter impregnated with (N-methyl-aminomethyl) anthracene (MAMA) for the vapour phase of isocyanates. This system effectively traps and separates the phases at the point of collection and offers many advantages over other methods for sampling isocyanates [SKC Iso-Chek 2017]. The principle of operation is described below. A sample pump draws air through the Iso-Chek cassette. Aerosols are trapped on the PTFE filter while gases pass through to the next filter. Vapours are trapped on the glass fibre filter impregnated with MAMA. A chemical reaction occurs on this filter resulting in the formation on a highly detectable urea derivative. The PTFE filter is derivatised in the field by placing it in a supplied jar containing 1,2-MP in toluene. Monomeric and oligomeric phases are separated by using a reverse phase HPLC column with a UVD and FLD in series.

However, the Iso-Chek method requires derivatization in the field, increasing the potential for sampling induced error, contamination, and under estimation if not immediately derivatized. The sampling media must be changed every 15 minutes, causing increased disruptions and lost productivity while outfitting the industrial worker. Moreover, the media requires stringent storage temperature and is relatively unstable with analysis recommended within 7-10 days.

4.2.2.3. Asset EZ4-NCO Method

Among the recently developed sampling devices, the Asset EZ4-NCO is the second commercial sampler and was put on the market as a method of reference for measuring the air concentration of the most commonly used isocyanates in the workplace [Sigma-Aldrich, 2013; Supelco Analytical 2013]. The sampler is a small solvent-free device that can be better adapted than an impinger to personal sampling. The Asset EZ4-NCO sampler is a tube in which its inner wall is covered with filter paper that is coated with a derivatisation reagent. A filter with the same derivatisation reagent is also added after the denuder to collect constituents that could have passed through the denuder. As the isocyanates are aspirated through the denuder, they are stabilised by the derivatisation reagent dibutylamine (DBA) that comes in contact with them, and this allows sample analysis in the laboratory. The combination denuder/filter impregnated with DBA used in the Asset EZ4-NCO sampler provides the same collection efficiency range as the impinger/filter approach for several applications involving isocyanate vapour forms [Marand et al., 2005; Nordqvist et al., 2005]. The unique design and the ease of use of the new dry sampling device present several advantages over existing devices such as the collection of both vapour phase and particulate isocyanates in one device; reliability – fast derivatization reactions into stable derivatives; complete derivatisation of particles; sampling for > 8 hours; no field handling of solvents or field desorption; and low detection limits of 50 - 100 times below existing methods. The new sampling devices will derivatise both the isocyanate monomers and oligomers. Selective determination of the urea derivatives is performed using LC-MS or LC-MS/MS.

However, sample preparation of the Asset EZ4-NCO is quite involved. It is targeted analysis rather than total isocyanates. Prior knowledge of the composition is required for the analysis of LC-MS/MS.

4.3. Critical Areas to Focus on Improvement of Methods

Selection of the most appropriate sampling and analytical method for quantitative monitoring of isocyanate exposure in a workplace environment is difficult for the following reasons: (1) isocyanates may be in the form of vapours or aerosols with various particle sizes; (2) the species of interest are reactive and unstable; (3) commercially available pure analytical standards are not available for all oligomeric isocyanates of interest and (4) low limits of detection are required. At the same time, efforts have been made to develop new sampling devices, derivatising reagents, and analytical methods with lower detection by many research groups across the world.

4.3.1. Sampling of Isocyanates (Impinger vs Filters)

Current glass impinger and filter cassette sampling methods present several challenges to researchers and occupational hygienists, such as sample collection efficiency, selectivity and sensitivity, and shipping compliance issues.

It is well known that the impinger approach has severe limitations. Risk of explosion is associated with this sampling device when it is used with a volatile solvent such as toluene. Potential leakages may occur during sampling in the personal breathing zone. Finally, the risk of flask breakage leading to solvent spill is an additional issue with this sampling device. The alternatives to impinger flasks are to use dry samplers, for example, filters impregnated by a derivatising reagent. There have been many efforts to use filters in the sampling of isocyanates as discussed above, but filters have a few disadvantages compared with impinger flasks for isocyanate sampling. Interference would affect more of the collection of an impregnated filter without solvent, and the reagent depletion on the filters would occur if the particle load were high. As a result, losses of isocyanates during sampling and underestimation of air concentration would become inevitable.

For several decades, studies have investigated alternative sampling techniques that would avoid the limitations linked to the use of impingers whilst offering the same sampling efficiency. Numerous studies have compared sampling results obtained using the methods discussed above, each with varying recommendations on individual method performance [England et al., 2000a and b; Carlton and England, 2000; Rudzinski et al., 2001; Rando et al., 2001; Thomasen et al., 2011; Ceballos et al., 2011; Reeb-Whitaker et al., 2012; Puscasu et al., 2014, 2015a and b, 2017, Aubin et al., 2020a and b]. The detailed discussions are given below.

The first commercially available sampler without using an impinger is Iso-Chek sampler. It has been selected as a primary sampling method in recent studies due to its ability to sample both monomeric and oligomeric isocyanates in the vapour and aerosol phases on a cassette.

One comparison study was conducted on airborne MDI concentrations associated with the application of polyurethane spray foam in residential construction. The results show that the impinger sampling method using impingers containing 1,2-MP in toluene [NIOSH 5521; HSE MDHS 25. 2014] gave higher airborne MDI and MDI oligomers concentrations than did the Iso-Chek [Lesage et al., 2007].

Another study critically compared 13 different air samplers for their ability to monitoring air exposure to HDI in the automotive refinishing industry. The midget impingers with frit were used as reference samplers and it was found that the Iso-Chek underestimated HDI compared with impingers samplers [Thomasen et al., 2011].

The second commercially available sampler, without use of impinger or solvent free and filter-based is ASSET EZ4-NCO [Marand et al., 2005; Nordqvist et al., 2005; Sigma-Aldrich, 2013]. Asset EZ4-NCO was used to quantify MDI aerosols in an MDI spray foam environment, parallel to the 1,2-MP/toluene impinger reference method [NIOSH 5521; HSE MDHS 25. 2014]. The ASSET sampler significantly underestimated the levels of MDI monomer and oligomers when compared to the reference method [Puscausu et al., 2015b]. Moreover, the ASSET sampler seemed to be saturated at some point and this could lead to the divergence obtained when compared to the reference method. The Authors stated that even though the prototype of the ASSET sampler performed well with vapour or slow-curing isocyanate applications in past studies [Marand et al., 2005; Nordqvist et al., 2005], the present study showed important limitations in the sampling and analysis of MDI aerosols from spray application. These field comparison results demonstrate the importance of evaluating each new sampler for each isocyanate application prior to a formal worker exposure evaluation.

In summary, it should be noted that there is no generic sampler suitable for all applications. It means that the selection of the sampling method will affect the results of the study. It is widely believed that the impinger-filter method is the most suitable method for sampling the potentially high concentrations of isocyanates in air. Furthermore, a combined denuder/filter sampler and Asset EZ4-NCO is a more valuable tool for the simultaneous determination of aerosols and vapour isocyanates than HSE MDHS 25 and Iso-Chek samplers.

4.3.2. Derivatisation

A very sensitive and selective analytical method is required for the identification of the specific isocyanate sensitising agent whilst monitoring it at very low concentrations and short exposures. Most analytical methods for isocyanate analysis rely on a derivatising reagent. The purposes of the derivatising agents are to: (1) react with isocyanates and form a stable urea derivative, and (2) improve analytical detection of isocyanates by strong molar absorptivity that increase sensitivity, or the limit of detection. In most cases, the combination of an impinger with a reagent-coated filter in series will collect both isocyanate aerosols and vapours efficiently. Some common derivatising reagents are summarised in Table 4.3 along with their suitable determination methods used for sampling isocyanates in air.

Table 4.3. Summary of the Derivatisation Reagents and Suitable Determination Methods Used for Sampling Isocyanates in Air

Derivatisation Reagent	Sampling	Analysis	References
1-(2-pyridyl)piperazine (1-2PP)	GFF	HPLC-UVD	OSHA 42/47 OSHA 5002
p-nitrobenzyl-N-propylamine (Nitro reagent)	Glass wool coated	HPLC-UVD or FLD	NIOSH 2535
1-(2-methoxyphenyl) piperazine (1,2-MP)	Impinger	HPLC-UVD or ECD	NIOSH 5521
3-(2-aminoethyl)indole (tryptamine)	Impinger	HPLC-UVD or ECD	NIOSH 5522
1-(9-anthracenylmethyl) Piperazine (MAP)	Impinger + Filter impregnated	HPLC-UVD/FLD	NIOSH 5525
1-(2-methoxyphenyl) piperazine (1,2-MP) 9-(methylaminomethyl) anthracene (MAMA)	PTFE filter + GFF filter impregnated	HPLC-UVD/FLD	Iso-Chek
1-(2-methoxyphenyl) piperazine (1,2-MP)	Impinger + Filter impregnated	HPLC-UVD/ECD	HSE MDHS 25
Dibutyl amine (DBA)	(GFF + denuder) impregnated	HPLC-MS or MS/MS	Asset EZ4-NCO
1,8-diaminonaphtalene (DAN)	CIP-10M	LC-MS/MS	Bello et al. 2005 Puscasu et al. 2016/2017

Among these derivatising reagents, 1-(9-anthracenylmethyl)piperazine (MAP) used in NIOSH Method 5525 has two important characteristics. The novel reagent was studied to show better sensitivity and selectivity, greater uniformity in the UV response across different isocyanate species, and improved reactivity compared to the majority of commercial derivatising reagents [Streicher et al., 1996; Rudzinski et al., 1996]. Other advantages of MAP include the replacement of the electrochemical detector with a more robust fluorescence detector.

The other novel derivatising agent, 1,8-diaminonaphtalene (DAN) has been developed recently for the total reactive isocyanate group (TRIG). Unlike most methods for isocyanate exposure, this evaluation use a reaction between an amine and the isocyanate function group to form a urea derivate, DAN, and applies this reaction as well to stabilise the isocyanate function group during field sampling. However, the DAN method has the unique characteristic in which during subsequent laboratory workup, an acid-catalysed cyclisation reaction produces one molecule of perimidone for each isocyanate group. The group subsequently is analysed by LC-MS/MS. This reaction offers several advantages for exposure evaluations targeting TRIG rather than separate monomer and oligomer species.

The derivatising reagent, 1,2-MP is probably the most commonly used reagent for the derivatisation of airborne isocyanates [Henneken et al., 2007]. However, piperazine compounds were declared controlled substances in 2013 in the UK as these compounds are used in the manufacture of illegal designer drug formulations and therefore cannot be used in impinger solutions for wet samplers or in the back section of impregnated filters for sampling isocyanates.

The field comparison study between Asset-EZ4-NCO and Iso-Chek was conducted [Aubin et al., 2020a and 2020b]. It is noted that the Asset EZ4-NCO uses a single DBA Dderivatising reagent whilst the Iso-Chek uses both 1,2-MP and MAMA derivatising reagents. The study was conducted on site comparing OSHA 42, Asset EZ4-NCO, Iso-Chek, DAN and CPI methods for measuring TDI at a polyurethane foam factory. It is found the Asset EZ4-NCO is more accurate than the Iso-Chek sampler [Aubin et al., 2020a]. These same samplers, including Asset EZ4-NCO and Iso-Chek, were used to measure MDI levels in an oriented-strand board factory and it is found that Asset EZ4-NCO provided a small bias comparing to Iso-Chek [Aubin et al., 2020b]. Both cases indicate that the Asset EZ4-NCO is advantageous over the IsoCheck and the derivatising reagents played an important role in sampling isocyanates.

In summary, the Asset EZ4-NCO sampler uses DBA as a derivatising reagent and field studies of the sampler have shown its reliability. Its applications have been increasingly popular. CIP 10M applies DAN as a derivatising reagent and the laboratory research shows promising results, however, requires further field studies.

4.3.3. Monomers and Oligomers

It is well known that the amount of free monomer in commercial systems is negligible, usually quoted by the chemical suppliers as < 1% of the free monomer [Sparer et al., 2004; Cocker, 2007; Hu et al., 2017]. Foam formulations using MDI normally have a monomer content of 50% while the remainder is made up of polymeric MDI oligomer. Around the world most regulations only cover the monomer, however, both monomer and oligomers should be measured, particularly in relation to worker-related illnesses [Bello et al., 2004]. More HDI oligomers were detected than HDI monomer in the air sampling studies in motor vehicle repair shops [Fent et al., 2009a and b]. To measure not only the monomer, but also oligomers, in the workplace air concentration has become more prevalent after a recently developed sampling device, the Asset EZ4-NCO, was put on the market approximately 10 years ago [Marand et al., 2005; Nordquist et al., 2005; Puscasu et al., 2015b; Aubin et al., 2020a and 2020b].

4.3.4. Detection

After reacting with the derivatising agent, the isocyanate derivative is usually analysed by HPLC in combination with UV/FL detectors or UV/EC detectors. Nowadays, a mass spectrometer is the preferred method for the detection of isocyanates from a range of different matrices. UV detector has low sensitivity and is less selective. FL detector has higher sensitivity compared with the UV detector but not many derivatising reagents are suitable for detection by the FL detector. Although the EC detector has the highest sensitivity among these three detectors, this detector is more variable than the UV/vis detector [White, 2006] and has been used as a qualitative approach in the HSE MDHS 25/4. EC detector is not compatible with LC gradient elution and is especially sensitive to changes in mobile phase [Streicher et al., 2000] and the cleanliness of the samples injected.

In general, the above three detectors are much less sensitive and specific compared to LC-MS/MS. With this instrument, using electrospray ionisation technique, an intact molecular ion is generated and enters the mass spectrometer, and one gains specificity with the use of a triple-quadrupole mass analyser. In the triple quadrupole, the initial ion of interest is isolated, then fragmented in a collision cell, and then unique ion fragments of interest are used to quantify the compound and confirm identity. In this MS/MS operation, signal-to-noise levels are increased dramatically by the reduction of noise. As a result, LC-MS determinations usually exhibit lower limits of quantitation (LOQ) than UV, FL and EC determinations. These lower LOQs are important for the detection of isocyanate oligomers in the air.

One disadvantage of the LC-MS/MS method in comparison to the LC/UV/EC method is that some prior knowledge of the composition is required before MS quantitation parameters are set. Another disadvantage of the LC/MS/MS method is the cost of the purchase and maintenance of an instrument and the analysis using LC-MS/MS also needs an analytical chemist with relatively high qualifications [White et al., 2012].

The LOQ for Asset EZ4-NCO and Iso-Chek methods are approximately an order of magnitude higher than the HSE MDHS 25 method (Table 4.2). Asset EZ4-NCO and Iso-Chek are equivalent on quantitation limit. However, Iso-Chek has a limited sampling time of 15 minutes while Asset EZ4-NCO is able to sample much longer at around 8 hours (480 minutes). This advantage for Asset EZ4-NCO makes it more sensitive than the Iso-Chek sampler.

4.3.5. Continuous Monitoring Exposure Isocyanates Techniques

Impinger and filters are the primary two sampling devices to collect aerosol and vapour isocyanates in the air. But so far, there are limitations in terms of efficiency or a lack of characterisation, especially for MDI during spray foam insulation application [Lesage et al., 2007; Puscasu et al., 2017]. To address these issues, a new approach using CIP 10M has been developed to MDI aerosols [Puscasu et al., 2015a].

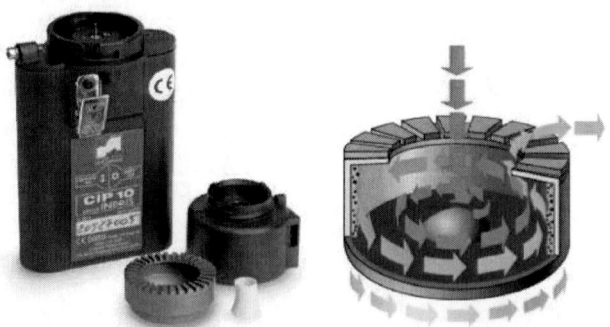

Figure 4.2. CIP 10 (CDL, carrefour du laboratorie) air sampler and the polyurethane foam creates the air flow and collects the dust.

The CIP10M is a commercially available personal aerosol sampler that has been validated for collection of microbial spores into a liquid medium (Figure 4.2). For use in sampling MDI aerosols (impinger), the aqueous medium normally used with CIP 10M has been replaced a non-volatile co-solvent in which the derivatisation agent 1,2-MP is introduced. Parallel sampling was performed in a real MDI foam spraying environment with a CIP 10M and impingers containing toluene/1,2-MP (reference method). The results obtained show that the CIP10M provides levels of MDI monomer in the same range as the impingers, and higher levels of MDI oligomers [Puscasu et al., 2015a].

There is another example of the application (filter) of CIP 10M in field evaluation of exposure to MDI vapour and aerosol in a real workplace using MDI-based spray foam. Both CIP 10/DAN and CIP 10/MP methods have lower detections of MDI compared to the reference method (a 13 mm filter coated with 1,2-MP). The study indicates that CIP 10 efficiently collected MDI vapours and particles below $1\mu m$. Comparing the impingers and filters approaches, no sampling pumps are needed as the CIP 10M has its own motor [Puscasu et al., 2017].

A recent study on site comparison of the five samplers including CIP 10 for measuring TDI at a polyurethane form factory was conducted and found that the CIP 10 method demonstrated a clear underestimation with large bias [Aubin et al., 2020a]. The most likely explanation was that the type of TDI emission was very poorly collected by the CIP 10 centrifugation mechanism. When the above samplers were used to measure MDI levels in an oriented-strand board factory, it is found that CIP 10 showed an underestimation with a large bias [Aubin et al., 2020b]. The same explanation given above for TDI most likely applies.

Nevertheless, CIP 10M seems to be a promising approach for isocyanate exposure evaluation in certain applications but many more studies need to be done. These studies and discoveries on selection of the most appropriate sampling and analytical method for quantitative monitoring of isocyanate exposure in a workplace environment demonstrate the need for a more in-depth investigation of the mechanism of collection, derivation, and analysis.

In summary, the Asset EZ4-NCO sampler (combined denuder/filter) is a valuable tool for simultaneous sampling and analysis of aerosols and vapour isocyanates in which DBA as the derivatization agent and MS/MS as the analytical approach are used. Although sampled isocyanates are generally analysed by HPLC coupled to UV, FL or/and EC detection, MS/MS detectors are preferred in particular when analysing isocyanate oligomers, due to better selectivity and sensitivity.

4.4. Occupational Exposure to Isocyanates

With the uses of developed and validated sampling and analytical methods for the determination of isocyanates and their oligomers, occupational hygienists and laboratory chemists are able to monitor worker's exposure to these toxic chemicals in their workplace. As discussed previously, no method from NIOSH, OSHA, HSE, or commercial companies is dominated in the field sampling and laboratory analysis, so occupational hygienists have to select the method depending on the workplace environment, or the industry groups as well as work area groups.

Unless stated otherwise, the exposure levels shown in this paper are given in the same metrics as in the original sources. For most of the data, exposure values refer to the measured masses (concentrations) of the respective monomers. However, since the NCO unit is assumed to be the toxicologically relevant functional group, it is difficult to compare exposure data for the different species (MDI, TDI, and HDI) and, if applicable, their polyisocyanates as such [Bello et al., 2004]. For direct comparison of exposure values of different diisocyanates in the discussion part, the units were therefore converted into 'total isocyanate group' values (μg NCO/m^3).

The potential for occupational exposure to isocyanates is determined by the intrinsic colligative properties of the substance (e.g., volatility) or by the processes involved in their handling [Rother and Schluter, 2011]. During the use of the various isocyanates products, occupational exposure can occur particularly for processes involving heating and spraying of isocyanates.

Activities such as hot wire cutting foams, welding through polyurethane pipe lagging, high temperature bonding using polyurethane sealants and hot removal of varnishes are activities that may lead to inhalation exposure to isocyanates. Very high exposures are found when a process is used where high levels of aerosols are formed (mostly spraying). Sanding of isocyanate containing materials such as paints, foams and plastics may also result in inhalation exposure from dust particles.

The Australian Workplace Exposure Study-Asthma, a national telephone survey, deemed that 2.5% of eligible participants were probably exposed to isocyanates at work in their current job (extrapolated to 3.0% of the Australian working population [El-Zaemey et al., 2018]. It is found that the most common tasks undertaken that led to these exposures were using expanding foam fillers/sprays and isocyanate and/or polyurethane paints. Exposure occurred mainly among construction workers, wood workers and painters or printers.

There are few peer-reviewed studies of workplace exposures to isocyanates in Australia. However, a study conducted in Western Australia of 25 motor vehicle repair shop workers showed no measurements of airborne concentrations above the LOQ of 0.1 NCO/sample [Hu et al., 2014].

Airborne isocyanate concentrations in overseas studies have been found to be generally very low (range 0.5-66 µg NCO/m^3). Creely et al., (2006) found a total 50 of the 70 samples they collected were less than 1 µg NCO/m^3, their LOQ for MDHS 25/3, hence assigned a value of half the LOQ (0.5 µg NCO/m^3). Of the 70 samples, 67 were below the UK TWA workplace exposure limit of 20 µg NCO/m3. The highest inhalation exposures occurred during spray painting activities in a truck manufacturing company (66 µg NCO/m^3) and during spray application of polyurethane foam inhalation (23 µg NCO/m^3).

Hon et al. (2016) described historical TDI, MDI and HDI exposures in two of the largest provinces in Canada (Ontario & British Columbia) between 1981-1996. In total, 6,894 isocyanate measurements were analysed, the majority of which were below the LOD (79%). Overall, 8.3% of samples exceeded the ACGIH TLV-TWA of 0.005 ppm (0.42 µg NCO/m3 for TDI, 0.61 µg NCO/m3 for MDI & 0.41 µg NCO/m^3 for HDI). However, most of the samples (95%) were area samples as impinger methods were the only option at that time.

Rother and Scluter (2021) grouped exposure data for the European Union (EU) according to industry groups as well as work area groups. The following uses were particularly relevant for occupational exposure and therefore the focus of the assessment was laid on: manufacturing of isocyanates, use in manufacture of PUs and PU composite materials, use in manufacture of foam, use in spray foam applications, use in coatings, and use in adhesives.

4.4.1. Manufacturing of Isocyanates

The main process to produce isocyanates is the phosgenation of corresponding diamines. Due to the dangerous properties of these two starting materials themselves, the production processes are carried out under containment in a high-integrity closed system [Falcke et al., 2017]. As long as the production is run under operating conditions, occupational exposure to isocyanates at this stage is generally considered to be low compared with the uses covering the application phases. The exposure estimates of the isocyanate species for manufacturing of the isocyanates as taken from the CSRs (Chemical Safety

Reports) are in the following ranges: MDI: 5.6 – 29 µg/m³; TDI: 5 – 32 µg/m³; and HDI: 3 – 23.5 µg/m³. These ranges are based on 90th percentiles of occupational hygiene measurement data and cover all contributing scenarios within the manufacturing scenarios.

4.4.2. Applications in the Manufacture of PUs and PU Composite Materials

The production of PU materials is the predominant use of isocyanates and has by far the highest volume. MDI is the most used isocyanate species for the production of PU materials. Compared with MDI, TDI plays a subordinate role in the production of PU materials, except for the production of block foams.

Table 4.4 provides an overview of the inhalation exposure levels to MDI and TDI in the manufacture of PU materials. Most of the data were collected between 1986 and 1993 after which the rate of data collection reduced significantly.

Table 4.4. Occupational inhalation exposure levels of isocyanate species (µg/m³) for use of isocyanates in the manufacture of PUs and PU composite materials

	CSRs 90th perc. range Long term/short term	IFA 90th perc. range (mean)Long term	HSE Range Long term	Literature data Range (Mean/median)
MDI	2-38/3-76	<LOQ[a]-18.0 (Mean 2.3) (N = 559)	0.09-32.8 (N = 13)	• <0.03-3.3 (MEAN 0.7) • (N = 131) [1] • 0.042-7.8 (med. 3.7) • (N = 10) [2] • <1-7.2 (N = 70) [3] • <0.6-3.3 (N = 46) [4]
TDI	1-32/1-64	4.0-67.3 (Mean 1.3) (N = 293)	-	0.08-14.6 (med. 1.2-3.9) (N = 14) [2]

[a] LOQ was not further specified in the IFA (2010) report; [1] Kaaria et al., (2001b); [2] Sennbro et al., (2004); [3] Creely et al., (2006); [4] Brzeznicki and Bonczarowska (2015).

4.4.3. Applications in the Manufacture of Foams

PU foams are generally divided by their elasticity into flexible, semi-flexible, and rigid foams. Foams are also the largest market for PUs, with flexible foams being the largest part. Both MDI and TDI are used in the production of foams. Due to the relatively low vapour pressure of MDI, the range of inhalation exposure to MDI in the manufacture of foam are usually low, compared with TDI in the manufacture of foams. TDI is an important component in the production of flexible foams. HDI is not considered to be relevant for the manufacture of foams.

Table 4.5. Occupational inhalation exposure levels of isocyanate species ($\mu g/m^3$) for use of isocyanates in manufacture of foams

	CSRs 90th perc. range Long term/short term	IFA 90th perc. range (mean) Long term	HSE Range Long term	Literature data Range (Mean/median)
MDI	6-29/12-58	<LOQ[a]-4.2 (Mean 1.7) (N = 1013)	0.03-0.17 (N = 3)	• <0.6 (N = 26) [4] • <0.6 (N = 20) [5]
TDI	1–32/1–64	<1.3-72.8 (Mean 4.7) (N = 110)	0.06–9.0 (N = 14) [Short term: 1.37–45.0 (N = 13)]	• <0.2–230 (N = 96) [1b] • 0.08–39.9 (med. 1.2–31.4) (N = 140) [2] • 0.2–58.8 (med. 4.0–9.8) (N = 26) [4] • 0.2–58.9 (mean 3.6–26.3) (N = 20) [5] • 46.5–73.6 (med. 62.9)b, • 5.0–86.5 (med. 12.5)c [6] • <7.2–17.4 (N = 26) [7] • 4.2–142 (mean 31.1) (N = 21) [8] • <0.71 (49 workers) [9] • • 0.03–3.1 (5 workers) [10]

[a] LOQ was not further specified in the IFA (2010) report.
[b] Before Risk Management Measures (RMM) improvements.
[c] After RMM improvements; [1b] Kääriä et al., (2001a); [2] Sennbro et al., (2004); [4] Brzeźnicki and Bonczarowska (2015); [5] Świerczyńska-Machura et al., (2015); 6] Tinnerberg and Mattsson (2008); [7] Austin (2007); [8] Geens et al., (2012); [9] Gui et al., (2014); [10] Jones et al., (2017), levels given as total NCO ($\mu g\ NCO/m^3$).

Data from CSRs, IFA, HSE UK and literature for inhalation exposure to MDI and TDI during the manufacture of foams are presented in Table 4.5. Some attention should be given to the values from the study by Tinnerberg and Mattsson (2008), where workplace measurement data from 13 Swedish industry plants were compared for before and after the installation of technical measures to improve the progress to reduce occupational exposure. After the modernisation and improvements of the plants, the exposure levels were found to be around 80% lower compared with the levels before.

4.4.4. Applications in Spray Foam

As spray applications are linked to particularly high exposure levels, compared with uses that take place in technically controlled environments or where only low mechanic energies are applied and therefore no or very low aerosol formation is to be expected, this use is considered as a special case. According to information from literature and the registration dossiers, the only isocyanates used for spray foam applications is MDI. Table 4.6 summarises the inhalation exposure levels to MDI during spray foam applications based on data from CSRs, IFA, HSE UK, and found literature relevant to the topic.

Table 4.6. Occupational inhalation exposure levels ($\mu g/m^3$) for use of MDI in spray foam applications

	CSRs 90th perc. range Long term/short term	IFA 90th perc. range (mean) Long term	HSE Range Long term	Literature data Range (Mean/median)
MDI	6-29/12-58	<LOQ[a] (Mean 1.9) (N = 35)	0.03-200 (N = 8)	• 0.07–2.47 (N = 36) [10] • 10–570 (N = 61) [11] • 70–2050 (N = 13) [12] • 11–591 (med. 54.8) (N = 94) [13] • <LOQ–770 [14] • <4.6–410 [15] • 30–90 (experimental set) [16] • 0.9–123.0 (GM 13.8) (N = 62) [17]

[a] LOQ was not further specified in the IFA (2010) report; [10] Jones et al., (2017), levels given as total NCO (μg NCO/m^3); [11] Crespo and Galán (1999); [12] Lesage et al., (2007); [13] Roberge et al., (2009); [14] RPS (2014); [15] Robert et al., (2014); [16] Puscasu et al., (2015b); [17] Bello et al., (2019).

4.4.5. Applications in Coatings

Coatings are often applied to surfaces by spreading or by spraying, and during these applications, often aerosols are generated and/or splashes occur, it is therefore often linked to particularly high exposures in comparison to uses with no (or minimal) aerosols/droplet formation.

All the diisocyanate species covered in this assessment (MDI, TDI, and HDI) are used in coatings. Inhalation exposure to MDI as well as TDI during application of diisocyanates-containing coatings is found to be relatively low compared with systems based on the more volatile HDI. Table 4.7 summarizes the inhalation exposure levels to MDI, TDI, and HDI for use in coatings based on data from CSRs, IFA, HSE UK, and found literature relevant to the topic.

Table 4.7. Occupational inhalation exposure levels ($\mu g/m^3$) for use of isocyanates in coatings

	CSRs 90th perc. range Long term/short term	IFA 90th perc. range (mean) Long term	HSE Range Long term	Literature data Range (Mean/median)
MDI	6-29/12-58	<LOQ[a]-18.8 (Mean 2.4) (N = 685)	-	• 0.06-8.1 [10] • <0.6 (N = 20) [5]
TDI	1-35/1-70	<1.3-6.0 (Mean 1.3) (N = 809)	-	-
MDI	110-430	<2.3-12.0 (Mean 2.3) (N = 1221)	0.35-208 (N = 15) [Short term:0.82-245000 (N = 47)]	• 421–423 [10] • med. 133–716 (N = 153) [18] • 0.02–57.6[b] (med. 0.08–7.4) (N = 95) [19] • 0.003–179 (GM 3.2) (N = 88) [20] • 0.02–946.7[b] (GM 87.2) [21]

[a] LOQ was not further specified in the IFA (2010) report.
[b] Data are presented for monomeric HDI; [10] Jones et al., (2017), levels given as total NCO (μg NCO m−3); [18] Sparer et al., (2004); [19] Pronk et al., (2006a); [20] Fent et al., (2009a); [21] Bello et al., (2020).

4.4.6. Applications in Adhesives

PU adhesives are used in a broad scope of applications and products ranging from extremely stable and weatherproof woodworking and construction glues to bonding automotive parts. The adhesives can be two-component or one-component systems, which themselves can be solvent-based, water-borne (aqueous dispersions), or solvent-free (granulates, dry powders). They can be processed and/or cured at ambient temperatures or at elevated temperatures. With respect to potential exposure, it was shown that both the content of isocyanate monomers and the processing temperature have a significant impact on emissions [Cuno et al., 2015]. Table 4.8 provides an overview of the inhalation exposure levels to MDI, TDI, and HDI in the use of adhesives as given in the CSRs, the MEGA evaluations by IFA, and as published by Brzeźnicki and Bonczarowska (2015).

Table 4.8. Occupational inhalation exposure levels ($\mu g/m^3$) for use of isocyanates in adhesives

	CSRs 90th perc. range Long term/short term	IFA 90th perc. range (mean) Long term	HSE Range Long term	Literature data Range (Mean/median)
MDI	5-43/9-87	<LOQ^a-6.5 (Mean 2.8) (N = 533)	-	• 0.6-5.2 (N = 20) [4]
TDI	1–35/1–70	<1.3-48.2 (Mean 1.9) (N = 308)	-	-
MDI	-	<2.3 (N = 294)	-	• 0.8-1.0 (N = 20) [4]

^{a} LOQ was not further specified in the IFA (2010) report; [4] Brzeźnicki and Bonczarowska (2015).

4.4.7. Discussions

It should be emphasized that many commercial products are not only based on isocyanate monomers but can consist predominately of oligomers and/or prepolymers (e.g., in HDI- based coating systems). Nevertheless, the majority of available exposure data is based on the measurement of the respective isocyanate monomer, whereas the measurement of 'total isocyanate group' values [Bello et al., 2004] has only recently become more common. It is understood that the overall risk of exposure to isocyanates is likely to be underestimated if these are not included. However, as written above, most of the available measurement data are for monomeric species, thus the focus in this chapter is on these.

Grouping of the exposure data in a ranking order according to the reported bandwidths of inhalation exposure levels results in the following order, inhalation exposure levels to:

- HDI and its oligomers in coatings – from 0.003 up to 5566.3 μg/m^3 (90th percentile), total range: 0.003-245000 μg/m^3
- MDI in spray foam applications – from limit of quantification (L0Q) up to 2050 μg/m^3
- TDI in manufacture of foam-from LoQ up to 203 μg/m^3
- TDI in manufacture of PUs and PU composite materials—from LOQ up to 67.3 μg/m^3
- TDI in adhesives—from LOQ up to 48.2 μg/m^3
- MDI in adhesives—from LOQ up to 43 μg/m^3
- MDI in manufacture of PUs and PU composite materials—from LOQ up to 32.8 μg/m^3
- TDI in coatings—from LOQ up to From LOQ up to 35 μg/m^3
- MDI in manufacture of foam—from LOQ up to 29 μg/m^3
- HDI in adhesives—from LOQ up to 1.0 μg/m^3

The uses found to give rise to the highest inhalation exposure levels are HDI (and its oligomers) in coatings and MDI in spray foam applications. In both uses, the isocyanates resins are applied by spraying, confirming that high exposures are to be expected when isocyanates are applied in high energy processes and aerosols are formed. Relatively high inhalation exposure levels are also found for some uses of TDI such as in the manufacture of foam as well as in the manufacture of PUs and PU composite materials and, in parts, for the use in adhesives. The exposure levels of MDI, on the other hand, for all these uses are significantly lower. These findings are in line with the expectation that the use of less volatile isocyanates leads to lower inhalation exposure levels.

While for most of the discussed uses, the majority of the measured data were quite low (near or below the LOQ), it has to be stressed that measurement of airborne isocyanates is technically challenging. The target compounds are usually highly reactive, and some measurement methods are less sensitive to this, hence resulting in systematic underestimation of the actual exposure levels at workplaces [Streicher et al., 2000, 2002; Bello et al., 2004]. Relatively high exposure levels can also occur in use that appears to be well controlled at the first sight (e.g., TDI in adhesives). Such relatively high levels of inhalation exposure seem to occur in an unpredictable and unexplained manner in all sectors and uses. The situation is further complicated by the fact, that different air sampling methods exist that measure differently (only monomers or total isocyanate mass concentrations, etc.), making comparison of measurement values between different studies more difficult [Bello et al., 2004].

4.5. Conclusion and Future Research Goals

There is no definitive sampling method best suited for all isocyanate sampling operations as, arguably, each method has limitations. The impinger, filter or a combination method is still an essential method for sampling isocyanates in workplaces. Among these derivatising reagents,

DAN offers more advantages over others for exposure evaluation targeting TRIG rather than separate monomer and oligomer species. More attention should be paid to the development of monitoring isocyanate oligomers. The majority of applications use HSE MDHS 25 and ISO-Chek samplers across the globe but Asset EZ4-NCO sampler has gained popularity in recent times. CIP 10 sampler is still in research phase but what it delivers so far looks promising.

The research priorities for sampling and analytical methods for airborne monitoring of exposure to isocyanates are developing new derivatising agents and low detection LC-MS/MS. Air sampling methods need to become easier to use. The long-term goal is to replace impingers especially when for personal sampling. Oligomers and/or total isocyanates methods should be evaluated and improved further. The liquid chromatography-tandem mass spectrometry should be much more widely applied in isocyanate analysis for enhanced speciation and quantification.

Chapter 5

Biological Monitoring and Its Applications

5.1. Introduction

Biological monitoring in occupational safety and health is the detection of substances (biomarkers) in biological samples of workers, compared to reference values. This chapter is limited to isocyanate exposure.

Biological monitoring can help in exposure assessment of specific chemicals, characterisation of exposure pathways and potential risks. Biomarkers can detect the exposure, the effect, or reveal susceptibility. Biological monitoring may be interpreted at the group or individual level. The most common media are urine and blood. While multitudes of substances can be measured, there are still only limited numbers of validated methods and limited values with scientifically proven backgrounds. The first paper on occupational biological monitoring was published in the USA [Badham and Taylor, 1927].

Within the occupational context, biological monitoring may help assess actual work risk, whereas air monitoring alone may seriously underestimate the total uptake of certain substances [EU Commission, 2018]. Characteristics of biological monitoring and workplace air monitoring are summarised in Table 5.1 [Manno and Viau, 2010].

Table 5.1. Comparison of biological and workplace air monitoring

	Biological Monitoring	Workplace air monitoring
Quantifying	Internal dose	External dose
Absorption	All routes	Inhalation only
Confounders	Metabolic phenotype	Personal protective equipment, substances with similar structure/chemical properties
Standardisation	Difficult	Easy
Interpretation	Difficult	Moderately difficult
Measurement	Indirect (biomarkers)	Usually indirect (dangerous substance)
Ethical issues	Important	None
Variability	High	Usually low

Biological monitoring is one of the most effective methods for measuring certain chemicals. While the application of biological monitoring varies across different parts of the world, there is a consensus that it plays an important role to determine and manage chemical exposures to minimise health risks for employees, in order to meet both industry standards and legislative requirements. One area of application that this Chapter will focus on is the utility of biological monitoring with respect to isocyanates in the motor vehicle industry, particularly as it can assess both dermal and inhalation exposure. There is no one method for monitoring airborne contaminants that could be present in the workplace. It is important to identify the substances that may be present, including substances that may be formed in work processes, and understand the associated hazards. One simple method is safety data sheets, which may contribute to the sampling strategy. In some cases, safety data sheets only provide information regarding the major components and do not necessarily highlight the ones that may cause the most harm. For example, air sampling based on ingredients in the safety data sheet does not produce analytical procedures for material samples, relevant air samples or any biomarkers.

Another common method is to focus on chemicals that are listed in the Workplace Exposure Standards (WES) lists in Australia. While this list is quite extensive, it is far from including all workplace hazardous chemicals. Further, the WES values do not necessarily state limits of chemicals that would provide exposed workers with a safe working environment, as some may have been set on a pragmatic basis, and some workers may be more susceptible than others. A more accurate risk assessment would include biological monitoring used in conjunction with the Occupational Exposure Limit (OEL).

This field has been slowly growing for many years but has recently had a strong acceleration thanks to the progress of analytical techniques. From an occupational point of view, the lowering of the exposure limits in the use of personal protective equipment and the attention to skin absorbance has increased the importance of knowing the individual dose for each worker, and even the legislation has become aware of this need.

The Health & Safety Executive (HSE) in the United Kingdom (UK) carries out the analyses of biomarker samples on behalf of occupational health providers, hygienists, hospitals and HSE staff. Urinary isocyanates analysis is the most frequent biomarker test in the UK, consistent with the experience of the Australian SafeWork NSW laboratory services in the last decade.

5.2. International Approaches

The regulatory framework for biological monitoring varies between the major developed countries. However, there is a consensus that biological monitoring is compulsory for workers if they are significantly exposed to lead. For almost all other substances, biological monitoring is optional but, in some cases, strongly advised and it is used widely in practical occupational medicine.

Various countries have published their own lists of Biological Exposure Limit (BEL) or Biological Limit Value (BLV). The BEIs® developed by the American Conference of Governmental Industrial Hygienists and the Biological Tolerance Values (BATs) established by the German Research Foundation represent two popular and extensive lists of occupational exposure guidelines used in biological monitoring. The European Union, the UK, Japan and other countries have developed their own lists as well. Although there is a substantial agreement among these organisations on the basics, there are several important distinctions in the approaches taken in setting the guideline values. Among these variances are: the specification of the biological monitoring guidelines as ceiling or average values; whether carcinogens should be treated differently from agents with other toxic outcomes; the method of accounting for variability among individual workers; and the extent to which these guidelines should be extended to include specific biomarkers such as genetic markers, indicators of susceptibility, or indicators of early biological response [Morgan and Schaller, 1999].

In America, the federal Occupational Safety and Health Administration (OSHA) produces biological monitoring guidance values for lead, cadmium and chromium as part of the Permissible Exposure Limit (PEL) process. However, the American Conference of Governmental Industrial Hygienists (ACGIH) produces a more stringent list of biological monitoring guidance values known as BEIs® [ACGIH, 2022]. Although BEIs® do not represent a legal standard, the ACGIH is widely recognised as an important professional society of industrial hygienists that offers guidance for the interpretation of biological exposure data. The majority of states in America use the BEIs®, in whole or in part.

Germany has probably the most extensive system for applying biological monitoring and developing guidance. BATs are recommended by a scientific expert group of the Deutsche Forschungsgemeinschaft (German Research Foundation, DFG). They are updated annually and published with the Maximale Arbeitsplatzkonzentrationen (MAK) (maximum workplace concentrations) for occupational exposure [Commission, 2007]. The BATs are legally enforced by the Federal Ministry for Employment and Social Affairs as Technical Guidelines. For substances with proven dermal absorption under usual working conditions, biological monitoring is mandatory [TRGS 150].

In the UK, biological monitoring can be used as part of the Control of Substances Hazardous to Health (COSHH) regulations for either health surveillance (regulation 11) or exposure assessment (regulation 10). The UK's Health and Safety Executive (HSE) framework for biological monitoring suggests it should be used where dermal absorption can give rise to systemic toxicity or where control of exposure relies on personal respiratory protection, particularly when air sampling alone cannot determine the level of exposure. The HSE encourages the use of biological monitoring by both occupational hygienists and physicians; and has a preference for non-invasive sampling [HSE, 1977]. Rather than basing their standards on extensive health studies as with America and Germany, the UK approach is based on statistical analysis. Many of the biological monitoring guidance values published by HSE [HSE, 2005] are based on the 90th percentile of biological values found in workplaces with good control.

In the EU, several Council Directives deal with biological monitoring for selected chemicals. The Scientific Committee on Occupational Exposure Limits (SCOEL) now considers BLVs as part of its work proposing Indicative Occupational Exposure Limit Values (IOELVs). However, many EU countries have their own regulatory framework for airborne and biological monitoring guidance values.

For most chemicals, only exposure-dose and exposure-effect relationships are known [Manini et al., 2007]. In this case, it is possible to identify the "mean" level of a biological index in a group of subjects exposed to air concentrations corresponding to the OEL for a given chemical. Many SCOEL BLVs are obtained from the corresponding OELs. Similarly, the BEIs® from the ACGIH is derived from corresponding Threshold Limit Values (TLV®), with a few exceptions. As a result, the interpretation of biological monitoring results between different countries is possible at the group level only. The German BATs of the DFG are between BEIs® and the health-based BLV standards. BATs are related to the maximum concentrations admissible in the workplace (MAK). They are also defined as "the maximum permissible quantity of a chemical substance or its metabolites or the maximum permissible deviation from the norm of biological parameter induced by these substances in humans" [DFG, 2022]. BATs are conceived as ceiling values for healthy individuals and "are intended to protect employees from impairment of health at work" [DFG, 2022]. As a result, BATs are expected to be higher than BEIs® values. Table 5.2 summarises and compares the characteristics of some biological values in terms of their origin and interpretation.

Table 5.2. Comparison among different biological limits, i.e., BEIs® (ACGIH), BATs (DFG), and BLV (SCOEL), in terms of their origin and interpretation

	BEIs (ACGIH)	BATs (DFG)	BLV (SCOEL)
Origin	Exposure-dose	Dose-response or exposure-dose	Dose-response (OEL-dose)
Corresponds to interpretation Criterion	Mean value Groups TVL-related	Ceiling values individuals or groups Health-based or MAK-related	NOAEL, ceiling values individuals and groups health-based
Carcinogens	Yes	No (EAK)	No

In Australia, the Work Health and Safety Act (WHS) places a duty on the person conducting a business or undertaking (PCBU) to ensure, so far as is reasonably practicable, the health of workers is monitored to prevent illness or injury. The WHS Regulations place specific duties on a PCBU to provide health monitoring to workers who use hazardous chemicals. The WES is a mandatory legal limit that must not be exceeded under the WHS Regulations [SWA, 2013]. The exposure standards state that airborne concentrations of individual chemical substances in the worker's breathing zone should not cause adverse health effects nor cause undue discomfort to nearly all workers, and establish a statutory maximum upper limit [SWA, 2013]. However, one drawback to this is that natural biological variation and the range of individual susceptibilities mean some people might still experience adverse health effects below the exposure standard, so the exposure standards do not necessarily represent an acceptable level of exposure to all workers. Australia's WES was first set by the National Health and Medical Research Council in the 1980s, based on ACGIH TLVs®. They were first published by SafeWork Australia's predecessor in 1990, the National Occupational Health and Safety Commission (NOHSC) [NOHSC, 1995]. Unfortunately, Safe Work Australia does not publish a list of BEIs®, although some guidance is available in the publication "Hazardous Chemicals Requiring Health Monitoring". It is recommended that biological exposure indices should either be adopted from the ACGIH BEIs® or the DFG BATs. Currently, the only biological exposure monitoring that is identified in the WHS regulations is for lead, although health monitoring is required for several substances.

The fundamental role of biological monitoring is to assess systemic uptake or exposure, in comparison with the different types of limit or guidance values, and link these data to biological effects. The combination of biological monitoring and health surveillance, as well as environmental monitoring, represent the fundamental tools for rational occupational risk assessment, as shown in Figure 5.1 [Mutti et al., 2006].

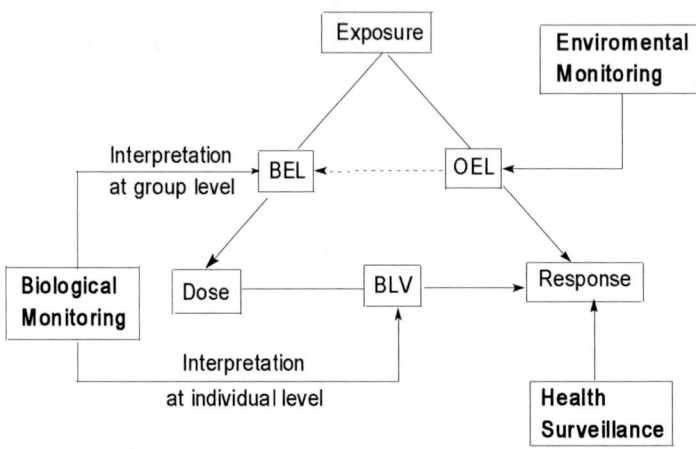

Figure 5.1. The link between external exposure, internal dose and biological response and their relationship with different types of occupational limit values (BEL, OEL, BLV). Modified from the "Guidelines on Biological Monitoring" of the Italian Society of Occupational Medicine and Industrial Hygiene [Mutti et al., 2006].

5.3. Assessing Exposure (Regulation)

Standards for acceptable levels of isocyanates range among different countries (Table 5.3). The German Commission for the Investigation of Health Hazards of Chemical Compounds in the Work Area has a Biologischer Leit-Wert (BLW) value for MDI of 10 µg MDA/L (4 µmol MDA per mol creatinine) based on the levels likely to be found in the urine after inhalation exposure to 50 µg MDI/m3 for eight hours [List, 2009].

Table 5.3. Reference values for assessing biological exposure to isocyanates

Biological level	Source
10 µg of methylenediamine (MDA)/L (~4 µmol MDA/mol creatinine) in urine	German Commission for the Investigation of Health Hazards of Chemical Compounds in the Work area BLW value
5 µg of TDAs/g creatinine in urine 15 µg of HDA/g creatinine in urine	BEIs from ACGIH
1 µmol of isocyanate-derived diamine /mol creatinine in urine	BMGV from HSE

The ACGIH [ACGIH, 2022] has a Biological Exposure Index (BEI) for TDI (2,4- & 2,6-isomers) exposures of 5 µg/g creatinine (3 µmol/mol creatinine) of toluene diamine in urine; and a BEI for HDI of 15 µg/g creatinine (10 µmol/mol creatinine) of 1,6-hexane diamine, collected at the end of shift.

In 2005, the HSE published a BMGV for isocyanates of 1 µmol of isocyanates-derived diamine per mol creatinine in urine samples collected at the end of exposure [HSE, 2010]. The BMGV was based on the 90th percentile of biological monitoring data from workplaces with exposure to HDI, TDI, or MDI. It is not a health-based guidance value but one based on exposure control. Any results exceeding the BMGV should simply trigger an examination of exposure controls and work practice with the intent of reducing exposure. Table 5.3 shows values that should be used as a guide for assessing exposure to isocyanates when urine analysis for isocyanate metabolites is performed.

There is a substantial body of work demonstrating the utility of biological monitoring as a tool to assess exposure and the efficacy of controls, including how it can be used in assessing exposure to isocyanates in the workplace. Non-health-based biological monitoring guidance values are also available to help target when and where further action is required. Occupational hygienists will need to use their knowledge and experience to determine the relative contributions of different routes of exposure and how controls can be improved to reduce the risk of ill health [Cocker, 2011].

5.4. Advantages and Disadvantages of Biological Monitoring

Biological monitoring has many advantages compared to air monitoring alone. Air monitoring can be used to estimate the inhalation (or dermal, etc) dose, which could be absorbed by workers. However, monitoring exposure through measurements of air levels may be difficult. For example, when assessing spray painters, air levels vary significantly with time. Also, some methods require complex equipment such as impingers; and may be unsuited to personal monitoring. Also, highly reactive air contaminants may have very short holding times prior to the required analysis. Such factors may affect the reliability of air monitoring results and may not give a relevant picture of the real short- or long-term systemic dose. A major advantage of biological monitoring is that all routes of exposure are taken into account. The sampling process does not interfere with everyday work tasks and also can be obtained after work has finished. Further, the number of samples that can be taken over a certain time period is greater for biomarkers than if air samples were used. This is because biological monitoring is more cost-effective and less intrusive for the workplace. Biomarkers can reveal the efficiency of personal protective equipment (PPE) worn or used by the workers, whereas air samples are taken outside of the PPE and, where respirators are used, do not reveal the worker's actual exposure. Air samples are much more prone to contamination during sampling as well. Biological monitoring is a more robust assessment method.

Another major advantage of biological monitoring is that it can measure the internal dose of hazardous workplace chemicals. Inhalation is often the major route of exposure at a workplace, with chemicals inhaled in the form of gases, vapours, liquid aerosols, dust, fumes or mixtures of these. Dermal uptake is also of concern, where exposure through the skin may occur from chemicals present in the air, form liquid splashes, through immersion, or handling of materials. Internal doses, which may be from multiple exposure routes, could lead to the development of disease and can be measured by biological monitoring for early intervention [Klaassen et al., 2001].

Air monitoring exposure to isocyanates has been established for the last four decades and there are many of choices for sampling methods. Occupational Exposure Limits (OEL) for isocyanates are well established. Biological monitoring has been developed for the last 2 decades. While biological monitoring has many strengths, its major weaknesses are that guidance values (for example, BEIs®), and there is potential for background levels or other source exposures.

Both air and biological monitoring are useful for the evaluation of occupational and environmental exposure to isocyanates. The toxic effect of the biggest concern related to exposure to isocyanate is occupational asthma. Therefore, the results of the determination of toxic isocyanates in the air are used for calculating toxic risk using the unit risk values.

Monitoring of airborne exposure to total isocyanate is costly, requiring considerable expertise, both in terms of sample collection and chemical analysis and cannot be used to assess the effectiveness of protection from wearing respiratory protective equipment (RPE). Biological monitoring by analysis of metabolites in urine can be a relatively simple and inexpensive way to assess exposure to isocyanates. It may also be a useful way to evaluate the effectiveness of control of measures in place.

Furthermore, common methods for the biological monitoring of exposure to isocyanates are based on the analysis of the amine derivatives in urine or blood samples after hydrolysis [Cocker, 2007; Tinnerberg et al., 2014]. This so-called 'total body burden' measurement does not distinguish between direct diamine exposure and diisocyanate exposure as analysis is based on the detection of the free diamine after hydrolysis of any diisocyanate conjugates. Because of the potential for confounding, this method may overestimate diisocyanate exposures because of other sources of free diamine. For example, in the case of MDI, methylene dianiline (MDA) is both a starting material for the production of MDI [Van Den Berg et al., 2012] and is an industrial chemical in its own right, used as a cross-linking agent for epoxy resins, as a corrosion inhibitor, as an antioxidant and curative agent in rubber, and to prepare azo dyes [NTP, 2021]. In addition, MDA exposure can also result from atmospheric hydrolysis of MDI during aerosol-generating activities such as spray painting and foam blowing [Jones et al., 2017].

5.5. Practical Approaches

5.5.1. Common Media

Most of the samples used for occupational safety and health are urine, blood, and exhaled air. There is a preference for non-invasive methods. Where available, such measurements may be used for screening and, if repeated at timed intervals, for monitoring either an individual or a group.

5.5.1.1. Urine
Urine is used for monitoring hydrophilic biomarkers of low molecular weight. Blood transfers the biomarkers from the absorption or metabolising sites to the kidneys, where they are excreted in the same way as endogenic metabolic waste. Urine collects in the bladder before it is voided; hence the concentration

of biomarkers in a urine specimen represents the average excretion during the interval between voidings.

The advantages of urine for biological monitoring are the non-invasiveness of sampling of sufficiently large samples and simple analysis that requires little clean-up procedures. The main disadvantage is that urine output, being influenced by water intake and loss (e.g., sweating, diarrhea), is highly carriable.

To eliminate the effect of fluctuating urine concentration being sampled, a practical means to normalise the results is to relate the excretion of the biomarker to the excretion of solids. Such adjustment can be either specific gravity (density) or creatinine excretion. The creatinine excretion rate in urine is more or less constant., and is independent of diet, hydration, and diuresis. This adjustment is not recommended if creatinine concentrations are outside the approximate range of 0.3-3.0 g/L because urine samples are considered "too diluted" or "too concentrated" [Viau et al., 2004].

5.5.1.2. Blood

Blood levels of parent compounds are the best indicators of internal exposure. However, the sampling of blood is considered invasive and can be done only by qualified personnel. Moreover, the analysis is usually complicated by a meticulous clean-up procedure. Blood is the only specimen available for measurement of macromolecular adducts, altered enzyme activity (cholinesterase), or some specific biomarkers resulting from the interaction of the pollutant with hemoglobin. Blood may be preferable for monitoring some metals and for monitoring poorly metabolised solvents, such as perchloroethylene.

5.5.2. Sampling

The concentration of isocyanates in the urine rises during exposure and is usually the highest in specimens collected at the end of the exposure. Biological monitoring for isocyanates has been available for many years [Rosenberg and Saviolainen, 1986 a and b] and is based on the analysis of isocyanate-derived diamines released by hydrolysis of protein adducts in urine or plasma. The dominant elimination half-lives of the isocyanates-derived diamines in urine are relatively short (2-5 hours), which means that urine samples should be collected at the end of exposure and the result mostly reflect exposure on the day collection. The longer half-lives of plasma adducts (20-

25 days) offer the potential for looking at integrated exposure over a longer period of time or investigating exposure incidents a short time after exposure has eased [Sennbro et al., 2004]. Recent work shows that methylene diphenyl diisocyanate (MDI) forms adducts with lysine in plasma albumin and may offer the potential for assessing risk [Sabbioni et al., 2010].

The test is easy to perform, requiring only a post-exposure urine sample. However, it is important that the sample, ideally, be taken within an hour of the end of exposure, especially for those tasks involving HDI, IPDI, and TDI. MDI exposure should be sampled at the end of the shift and, if significant skin exposure is possible, pre-shift next-day samples should also be considered (due to the delayed absorption through the skin). Because of the short half-life of excretion, the sample mostly reflects that day's exposure and so does not inform on long-term exposures. It is therefore recommended that several samples are taken initially to ensure that "normal" practice is captured. Samples should be sent the same day or the next day to a suitable laboratory for analysis. If shipping is delayed, samples should ideally be stored frozen prior to despatch [Jones, 2019].

5.5.3. Analytical Methods

Over the last three decades, multiple analytical methods have been developed for the measurement of urinary aliphatic and aromatic diamines. The majority of the methods involve acid or basic hydrolysis followed by liquid-liquid extraction and sample derivatisation steps prior to gas chromatography-mass spectrometry or liquid chromatography-mass spectrometry based on analysis.

Improvements in terms of ease, quickness, sensitivity, etc have been attempted in the steps of extraction, derivatisation, and detection technique for sample preparation.

5.5.3.1. Hydrolysis

The very first step of the sample preparation for the analysis of urinary isocyanate samples is the hydrolysis of urine under acidic or alkaline conditions (Tables 5.4 a, b, c). Over the last 30 years, laboratories applied various experimental conditions for the hydrolysis of urine.

The process involves heating the urine samples at a given time. The acids such as H_2SO_4 and HCl and basic such as NaOH have been used in hydrolysis. The experiments demonstrated both conditions are effective, but most applications have applied H_2SO_4 when the total concentration of urinary diamines is required. It is also found that too harsh hydrolysis conditions might lead to artifacts and too mild conditions might lead to small yields.

Upon exposure, isocyanates are converted *in vivo* to corresponding diamines. These diamines form conjugates with a variety of functional groups on macromolecules including, hydroxyl, sulfhydryl, and amino groups. In addition, diamines can undergo N-acetylation to form mono- and di-acetylated diamine metabolites, which are readily excreted in the urine. Acid hydrolysis of urine can break down both conjugated and acetylated diamines into a free form while base hydrolysis is only effective for conjugated diamines.

It was reported [Cocker et al., 2017] that using alkaline hydrolysis encountered high 'background' levels in the HDA analysis. It was not clear if the hydrolysis was producing HDA from endogenous substances or whether the interference was simply a co-eluting peak. This is perhaps why acid hydrolysis is preferred over base hydrolysis as acid hydrolysis minimises the interference.

It is also found from the same study [Cocker et al., 2017] that in many isocyanate-containing products, particularly HDI, the isocyanates are present as oligomers or polymers with little free isocyanate monomers. If the levels of HAD found in urine seemed to be higher than might be expected from exposure to just the HDI monomers, this may suggest that the hydrolysis is releasing HAD from some of the oligomeric HDI-Conjugates.

5.5.3.2. Extraction

The extraction of hydrolysed compounds in urine samples can be performed using liquid-liquid extraction with toluene [Marand et al., 2004, Skarping et al., 1994], dichloromethane [Sakai et al., 2002], ethyl ether [Williams et al., 1999], or using a solid-phase extraction [Bhandari et al., 2016, 2018] (Tables 5.4 a, b, c).

After hydrolysis, amines in urine samples that are corresponding to isocyanates derived from metabolites are released. Due to their relative polar property in aqueous solution, a non-polar solvent such as toluene is often used, which is often called liquid-liquid extraction. In the early studies, toluene has been used due to its property close to those of aliphatic and aromatic amines. However, two other solvents have been used, diethyl ether for HDA extraction [Williams et al., 1999] and dichloromethane for HDA oligomer [Robbins et al., 2018], for MDA [Kaaria et al., 2001b], and for TDA [Sakai et al., 2002] extractions, respectively. The use of toluene rather than dichloromethane as an extraction solvent is a small advantage as it allows the collection of the top layer.

Apart from liquid-liquid extraction, solid-phase extraction has been also used in this step, especially in recent studies [Bhandari et al., 2016 and 2018, Lepine et al., 2020].

The solid-phase extraction method has been using reversed-phase material for 100 years. Reversed-phase SPE separates analytes based on their polarity. The stationary phase of a reversed-phase SPE cartridge is derivatized with hydrocarbon chains, which retain mid to low polarity compounds due to the hydrophobic effect. The analyte can be eluted by washing the cartridge with a non-polar solvent, which disrupts the interaction of the analyte and the stationary phase.

In the last decades, ion exchange sorbents have been introduced. The sorbents separate analytes based on electrostatic interactions between the analyte of interest and the positively or negatively charged groups on the stationary phase. For ion exchange to occur, both the stationary phase and sample must be at a pH where both are charged. The combination approach of reversed-phase and ion exchange in SPE is called mixed-mode.

LLE has the advantages of low cost, short procedural time, and low method detection limit. However, SPE provides several advantages over LLE including higher recoveries, elimination of emulsion, less organic solvent usage, easier operation and possibility of automation, improved selectivity and reproducibility and shorter sample preparation time. The extraction process is more selective when mixed-mode exchange sorbent is used comparing the traditional C18 sorbent and liquid-liquid extraction approach.

In 2016, Bhandari et al., first applied the SPE approach to the determination of the measurement of aromatic diamines in urine in the sample preparation step. The SPE was performed here because of the advantage of strong cation-exchange-, π-π interaction-, and hydrophobic-interaction-based mechanisms offered by a mixed mode strong cation exchange cartridge. These aromatic diamines such as TDA and MDA should be positively charged at a pH 2 according to Henderson-Hasselbalch approximation. Therefore, below pH 2.4, maximum recovery is expected for these diamines, which are primarily retained by the SPE sorbent through electrostatic interactions.

In 2019, a similar SPE method was applied to the determination of both aliphatic (HDA) and aromatic diamines (TDAS and MDA) in urine [Lepine et al., 2020]. The SPE sorbent is a mixed-mode cation exchange polymer cartridge that is less strong than the one used in the studies for aromatic diamines in urine [Bhandari et al., 2016].

Another method for the determination of both aliphatic and aromatic amines as Acetic anhydride derivatives in urine samples using liquid chromatography and tandem mass spectrometry has been developed recently, in which solid phase extraction was used rather than a liquid-liquid extraction approach [Lepine et al., 2020]. Its sample preparation is briefly described below: At first, an internal working solution was spiked into urine samples, followed by the addition of sulphuric acid. The mixture was heated overnight and cooled to room temperature followed by the addition of NaOH and centrifuged to remove an insoluble material prior to solid-phase extraction. SPE was performed using mixed-mode cation exchange cartridges. After conditioning the cartridges, samples were then loaded on the cartridges, methanol was added to wash the cartridges. The sample was eluted using NH_4OH containing methanol. Eluents were then evaporated to dryness. Extracts were reconstituted with borate buffer and instantly derivatised with the addition of pure acetic anhydride at room temperature. Samples were finally centrifuged to remove any insoluble material and transferred to a vial with an insert for LC-MS/MS.

In Bhandari's study, it is the first time that an automated solid phase extraction (SPE) was applied in the sample preparation. The replacement of liquid-liquid extraction (LLE) used in almost all methods in the literature for sample preparation has made the method straightforward, fast, and well-suited for high-throughput clinical and research laboratories.

5.5.3.3. Derivatisation
After hydrolysis and extraction, the yielded diamines were derivatized with heptafluorobutyric acid anhydride (HFBA) [Cocker et al., 2017; Lewalter et al., 2000; Sabbioni and Beyerbach 2000] or pentafluoropropionic acid anhydride (PFPA) [Sennbro et al., 2003; Sennbro et al., 2005] for all GC-MS methods and with HFBA for one LC-MS/MS method [Marand et al., 2004]. For the LC-MS/MS method by Lepine et al. [Lepine et al., 2020], the extracts were derivatized with an acetic acid anhydride. The LC-MS/MS method of Bhandari et al. [Bhandari et al., 2016] for the analysis of MDA, 2,4-TDA, 2,6-TDA, NDA, and 1,4-PDA was performed without prior derivatization. This is also the case for the analysis of MDA by Lepine et al. [Lepine et al., 2019].

The amines such as TDIs and HDA are more polar molecules, making their analysis by reverse-phase LC-MS challenging, especially in a complex matrix such as urine. Derivatisation is necessary to have appropriate chromatographic retention and sensitivity for TDA isomers and HDA for both GC-MS and LC-MS (Tables 5.4 a, b, c).

Acetic anhydride was used recently [Robbins et al., 2018, Lepine et al., 2020] because it was known to yield a simple and fast reaction with free amines [Baker et al., 1994] without the need to remove excess reagents like HFBA and PFPA.

One of the drawbacks of the above analytical approaches using either GC-MS or LC-MS method is a time-consuming procedure with complicated derivatisation. On the other hand, the derivatisation step is a time-consuming procedure. An effort to avoid this procedure has been attempted. Sakai made the first report in 2002 on the direct determination of urinary TDAs without derivatisation using the LC-MS method. The application of the LC-MS method in the report reduced the cycle of analysis by half compared with those using the GC-MS method. More recently, two LC-MS/MS methods [Bhandari et al., 2016 and Lepine et al., 2019] have been developed to analyse aromatic diamines in human urine in which the sample preparation procedures are not involving derivatisation.

5.5.3.4. Detection

The LODs for the single diamines vary substantially between the methods (Tables 5.4 a, b, c) and the LODs or LOQ for each method in the Table are quoted as a reference or guide. For the practical purpose, the lowest LODs of methods that analyse at least 4 diamines were elucidated. The LODs decrease in the following order: [Marand et al., 2004], [Bhandari et al., 2016], [Cocker and Jones 2017], [Lepine et al., 2020].

The GC-MS method by Cocker and Jones [Cocker et al., 2017] was tested by other laboratories in the process of validation for the MAKcommission. The LC-MS/MS method by Hu et al. [Hu et al., 2017) which was modified from Marand [Marand et al., 2004] passed successfully the German External Quality Assessment Scheme (G-EQUAS, https://www.g-equas.de/) test for MDA, 24TDA, 26TDA, and HDA. The lower test concentration (G-EQUAS, 57/2016) for MDA, 2,4-TDA, 2,6-TDA, and HDA are 5.69, 3.65, 3.17, and 3.11, ng/mL respectively. Up till now, the lower test concentration (G-EQUAS, 69/2022) for MDA, 2,4-TDA, 2,6-TDA, and HDA are 5.69, 0.85, 0.69, and 2.53, ng/mL respectively. It can be seen that only concentrations for 2,4-TDI and 2,6-TDI have been dropped. In addition, other LC-MS/MS method [Lepine et al., 2020] was tested in an interlaboratory comparison or reviewed by external laboratories, passing successfully the G-EQUAS (66/2020).

Table 5.4a. The summary of developed analytical methods for the determination of HDI in urine samples

Method	Hydrolysis	Extraction	Derivatisation	Detection	LOD/LOQ (µg/L)
Rosenberg 1986a	H2SO4	Silica gel cartridges	HFBA	GC-MS	34
Brorson 1990	H2SO4	Toluene	HFBA	GC-MS	0.5
Dalene 1994a	NaOH or H2SO4	Toluene	Ethyl chloroformate	GC-MS	0.5
Skrpping 1994	H2SO4	Toluene	PFPA	LC-MS	0.5
Tinnerberg 1995	NaOH	Toluene	PFPA	LC-MS	0.1
Maitre 1996	HCl	Toluene	HFPA	GC-MS	1
Marand 2004	H2SO4	Toluene	PFPA	LC-MS/MS	0.5
Hu* 2014, 2017	H2SO4	Toluene	PFPA	UPLC-MS/MS	0.5
Cocker 2017	H2SO4	Diethyl ether	HFPA	GC-MS	0.2/0.7
Bhandari 2018	HCl	SPE (mixed-mode) cation exchange)	NA	UPLC-MS/MS	0.15
Robbins 2018	H2SO4	Dichloromethane	Acetic anhydride	UPLC-MS/MS	0.03
Lepine* 2020	H2SO4	SPE (mixed-mode cation exchange)	Acetic anhydride	UPLC-MS/MS	0.9

* Methods participated successfully in G-EQUAS.

Table 5.4b. The summary of developed analytical methods for the determination of TDI in urine samples

Method	Hydrolysis	Extraction	Derivatisation	Detection	LOD/LOQ (µg/L)
Sandstrom 1989	H2SO4	Toluene	PFPA	GC-MS	0.1
Brorson 1991	NaOH	Toluene	PFPA	GC-MS	0.1
Skrpping 1991	NaOH	Toluene	PFPA	GC-MS	0.1
Maitre 1993	HCl	Toluene	HFBA	GC-MS	0.1
Carbonnelle 1996	NaOH	strong cation exchange sorbent		LC-ECD	0.1

Method	Hydrolysis	Extraction	Derivatisation	Detection	LOD/LOQ (µg/L)
Lind 1996	H2SO4	Toluene	PFPA	GC-MS	0.15
Kaaria 2001a	H2SO4	Toluene	HFBA	GC-MS	0.1
Sakai 2002	NaOH	dichloromethane		LC-MS	1
Sennbro 2003	H2SO4	Toluene	PFPA	GC-MS	0.1/0.5
Marand 2004	HCl	Toluene	PFPA	LC-MS/MS	0.5
Bhandari 2016	H2SO4	SPE (mixed-mode strong cation exchange)	Nil	LC-MS/MS	0.03/0.1
Hu* 2014, 2017	H2SO4	Toluene	PFPA	UPLC-MS/MS	0.5
Cocker 2017	H2SO4	Diethyl ether	HFPA	GC-MS	0.1/0.4
Lepine 2020	H2SO4	SPE (mixed-mode cation exchange)	Acetic anhydride	UPLC-MS/MS	0.3

* Methods participated successfully in G-EQUAS.

Table 5.4c. The summary of developed analytical methods for the determination of MDI in urine samples

Method	Hydrolysis	Extraction	Derivatisation	Detection	LOD/LOQ (µg/L)
Tiljander 1989	H2SO4	Toluene	PFPA	GC-MS	2
Schutze 1995	H2SO4	Toluene	HFBA	GC-MS	2
Skarping 1995			HFBA	GC-MS	1
Kaaria 2001b	H2SO4	dichloromethane	HFBA	GC-MS	0.3
Sennbro 2003	NaOH	Toluene	PFPA	GC-MS	0.05/0.6
Marand 2004	H2SO4	Toluene	PFPA	LC-MS/MS	0.5
Bhandari 2016	HCl	SPE (mixed-mode strong cation exchange)	Nil	LC-MS/MS	0.01/0.03
Hu* 2014, 2017	H2SO4	Toluene	PFPA	UPLC-MS/MS	0.5
Cocker 2017	H2SO4	Diethyl ether	HFPA	GC-MS	0.1/0.4
Lepine* 2020	H2SO4	SPE (mixed-mode Cation exchange)	Acetic anhydride	UPLC-MS/MS	0.6

* Methods participated successfully in G-EQUAS.

5.5.4. Interpretation

In all cases, the reliability and validity of biological monitoring results should be ensured in the design and evaluation of the sampling strategy.

Factors influencing the reliability include: the day of the sampling not being representative of the usual occupational exposure, sampling time not appropriate according to exposure time, external contamination, inappropriate storage and transport conditions, as well as urinary creatinine levels out of 0.3 - 3.0 g/L.

Additionally, the identification of possible confounding factors include, for example, exposure due to non-occupational sources (e.g., food, smoking, drugs), diseases promoting metabolic disorder or excretion disturbance may have to be considered. The comparison of biological monitoring results can be done according to the following flow chart (Figure 5.2).

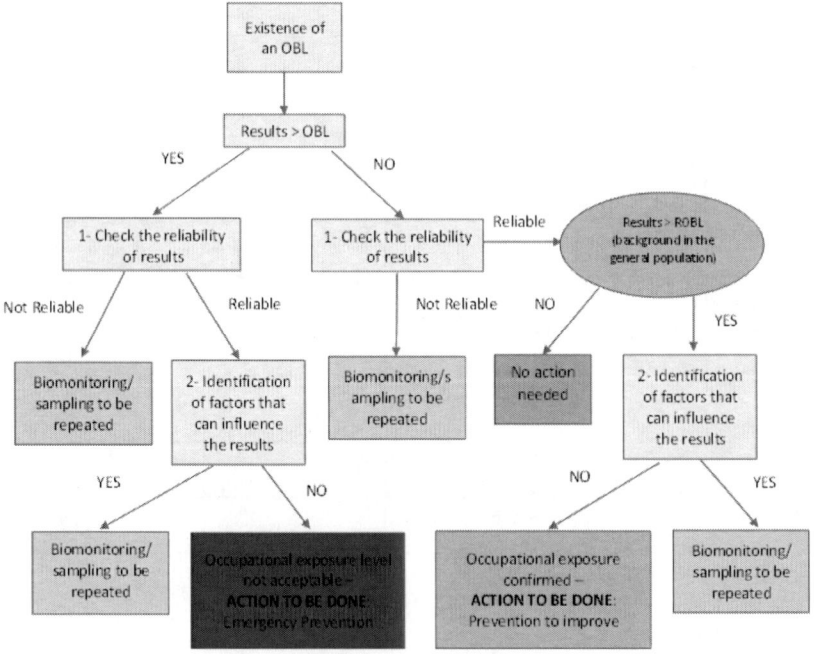

Figure 5.2. Interpretation of biological monitoring results, adapted from [SFMT, 2016].

Non-compliance with OBL is an indication of inadequate risk management measures. In addition to inadequate risk management measures, the following reasons for elevated biological monitoring values shall be considered:

- lack of compliance by individuals with personal hygiene requirements at work
- a specific co-exposure scenario that may affect the toxicokinetics of the biomonitoring parameter
- non-occupational exposures
- exposures that occurred a long time ago (for substances that accumulate in the body)
- individual health/medical conditions that influence substance uptake, excretion or metabolism.

In some cases, isocyanate-derived diamines, other than those expected, were found and reported. The subsequent investigations usually indicated previously unknown isocyanate exposure rather than analytical interference. The analytical method is intended to assess exposure to isocyanates but by measuring diamines in urine it will also detect any exposure to the diamines. Co-exposure to both isocyanates and diamines should be considered when interpreting results.

5.5.5. Criteria for Selection of a Biomarker

The selection of biomarkers, biological specimens, and the timing of sample collection depends on the purpose of the monitoring. For confirmation of overexposure, or for medical screening, measurement in a single sample collected during or after the exposure is suitable, provided that the biomarker still persists in the body. Samples collected within the period of three half-lives following exposure are usually timely. For retrospective verification of past exposure(s), biomarkers with long half-lives, such as macromolecular adducts, are suitable. For routine exposure monitoring and potential risk assessment, biomarkers that are excreted in the urine are the first choice, because of the convenience of urine sampling. For medical surveillance and health risk evaluation, biomarkers that are related to toxicology are preferable. However, further steps should be taken to identify the pollutant causing the health problem.

In selecting a biomarker for biological monitoring, the following factors should be considered: specificity of the biomarker; sensitivity and background level of the biomarker; availability of an analytical method; and stability of the sample and of the biomarker during storage and transportation.

There is no exception that the development of selecting a biomarker for biological monitoring exposure to isocyanates has been following the above rules. The development of analytical methods for the determination of amines in urines has been focused on individual amines, such as HDA for aliphatic amine or TDA and/or MDA for aromatic amine. HDA as a biomarker for HDI was first analysed in 1986 after hydrolysis, and silica gel extraction [Rosenberg and Saviolainen, 1986a]. TDI and MDI were first analysed in 1989 [Sandstrom et al., 1989] and in 1989 [Tiljander et al., 1989], respectively. A screening method for all amines in urine for both aliphatic and aromatic amines in urine was developed in 2004 [Marand et al., 2004] by LC-MS/MS and in 2017 by GC-MS [Cocker et al., 2017], respectively.

The isocyanate-protein adducts are sufficiently stable for the samples to be sent by post to the laboratory for analysis. The analytical methods are capable of detecting isocyanate exposure well below current occupational exposure limits. Because the analysis is based on the hydrolysis of conjugates, there is little risk of sample contamination during collection. However, any diamines present during exposure would also be detected and could lead to an overestimate of isocyanates exposure (Pauluhn and Lewalter, 2002). Urinary concentrations of toluene diamine (TDA), NDA, and MDA in people not occupationally exposed are 0.1 µmol/mol (Rosenberg et al., 2002; Sennbro et al., 2005).

After 30 years HDA was first analysed as a biomarker for occupational HDI exposure in 1986, the discovery of a new biomarker for monitoring exposure to isocyanates has been developed actively in the last decade, mainly due to the advances in LC-MS/MS technique.

Common methods for the biological monitoring of exposure to isocyanates are based on the analysis of the amine derivatives in urine or blood samples after hydrolysis [Cocker, 2007; Tinnerberg et al., 2014]. The use of hydrolysed diamines in urine as biomarkers of isocyanates has been widely adopted by international bodies setting guidance values [ACGIH, 2022; DFG, 2021; HSE, 2020]. This so-called 'total body burden' measurement does not distinguish between direct diamine exposure and isocyanate exposure as analysis is based on the detection of the free diamine after hydrolysis of any isocyanate conjugates. Because of the potential for confounding, this method may over-estimate isocyanate exposures because of other sources of free diamine.

A recent significant development in the analysis of diamines in human urine was to focus on the analysis of metabolites of isocyanate oligomers instead of monomers. Robbins [Robbins et al., 2018] first reported 2018 the determination of trisaminohexyl isocyanurate (TAHI), hydrolysis of the product of HDI isocyanurate (Figure 5.3), in the urine of spray painters. The method is sensitive and specific with a method limit of 0.03 µg/L. This new biomarker for HDI isocyanurate is believed to be critical to determine the relative potency and dose relationships between the monomer and oligomer exposure to the development of diisocyanate-induced health effects in future studies.

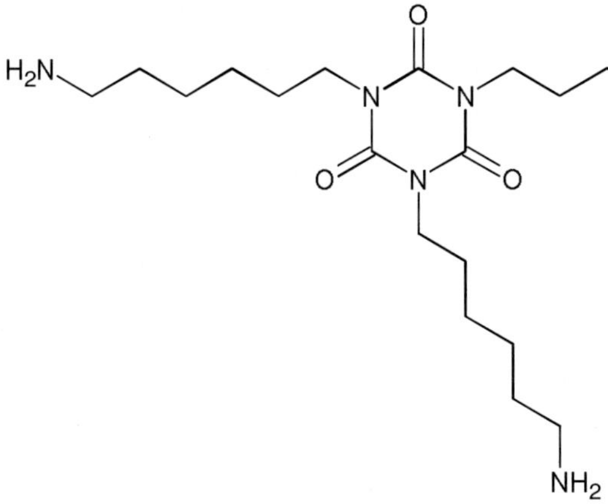

TAHI, FW: 426.6

Figure 5.3. Molecular structure of HDA Isocyanuarate as a biomarker for HDI Isocyanuarate.

The metabolism of isocyanates is not fully understood at present; however, MDI conjugation to human albumin in vitro has been reported [Wisnewsk1 et al., 2013]; a recent review [Schupp and Plehiers, 2022] has collated work in this area, outlining the known mechanisms of MDI absorption, distribution, metabolism and excretion and detected biomarkers (both in vitro and in vivo). Lysine residues have been reported as the predominant binding sites on human serum albumin (HAS) for TDI and MDI [Hettick and Siegel, 2012; Hettick et al., 2012; Mhike et al., 2013]. This knowledge has led to research into the discovery of new biomarkers of isocyanates exposure. A method to extract and quantify isocyanate-specific conjugates with albumin was first reported in rats [Kumar et al., 2009].

Sabbioni and co-workers built on this work and reported MDI specific HAS conjugates in plasma from exposed workers; acetylated MDI-lysine (acMDI-Lys) (Figure 4) and MDI-Lysine (MDI-Lys) conjugates were detected in exposed workers from a chemical company and a construction site. MDI-Lysine conjugates were found in over 60% of samples tested in both companies [Sabbioni et al., 2010]. The presence of the MDI-lysine conjugates in albumin isolated from human blood plasma samples of persons undergoing Specific Inhalation Challenge (SIC) for MDI was also reported [Sabbioni et al., 2016]. A separate study also reported MDI-Lys conjugates that were detected in MDI workers' sera samples after SIC for MDI [Luna et al., 2014].

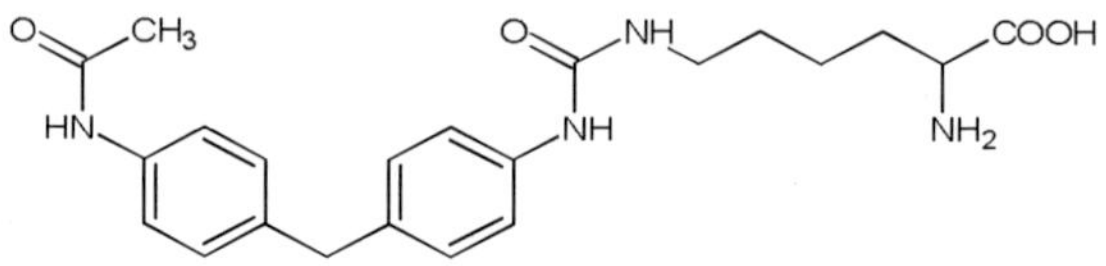

AcMDI-Lys, FW: 412.5

Figure 5.4. Molecular structure of acetyl-MDI-Lysine as a biomarker for MDI.

Given the invasive nature of blood sample collection and ethical considerations, an alternative analytical approach is desirable. Human biomonitoring or biological monitoring using urine samples offers many advantages. Urine is a primary excretory pathway, non-invasive, and a suitable matrix for the detection of a wide range of both organic and inorganic compounds and metabolites from occupational and environmental exposure [Polkowska et al., 2004; Smolders et al., 2009]. Despite these advantages, care needs to be taken in collecting the sample to avoid contamination (from skin or clothing) and to collect the sample at the right time post-exposure.

Specific urinary metabolites of MDI exposure have not yet been reported in humans, although detection of dilysine-MDI in the urine of MDI-exposed mice has been reported [Wisnewski et al., 2019]. An investigation [Wisnewski et al., 2022] explored the reactivity of glutathione (GSH) with aliphatic polyisocyanates most commonly used in industry today. LC-MS/MS was used to characterise reaction products generated under physiologic conditions and model their chemical structures. It is found that the aliphatic polyisocyanates readily react with GSH to form primary S-linked tris (GSH)-conjugates, a process that may play an important role in response to respiratory tract exposure.

The analysis of acMDI-Lys in the urine of workers exposed to MDI was first reported in 2022 [Nwoko et al., 2022], and acMDI-Lys may be a useful non-invasive biomarker in discriminating between MDI and MDA exposures. Urine samples were obtained from a group of workers exposed to methylenediphenyl diisocyanate (MDI) where aerosol generation was unlikely. Lysine conjugates of MDI were extracted from urine by solid phase extraction; analysis was performed by liquid chromatography-tandem mass spectrometry. Acetylated MDI-lysine (acMDILys) conjugates were detected in 73% of samples tested from persons with exposure to MDI compared to 93% of samples that were positive for methylene dianiline (MDA) in hydrolysed urine. There was a weak but significant positive correlation between the two biomarkers ($r^2 = 0.377$).

At the same time, a new discovery of the isocyanate adduct of HDI with lysine was reported [Sabbioni and Pugh, 2022]. The presence of HDI-Lys (Figure 5.5) was found after pronase digestion of albumin and confirmed by LC-MS/MS method for the analysis of HDI adducts in Vivo modified albumin and in workers. Quantification was performed and the adduct peak found in vivo was confirmed. This study indicates that increased levels of HDI-Lys might correlate with an increased risk of isocyanate occupational asthma and the new biomarker has the potential to establish a biological tolerance value (BAT-value) that prevents isocyanate-induced asthma [Sabbioni and Pugh, 2022].

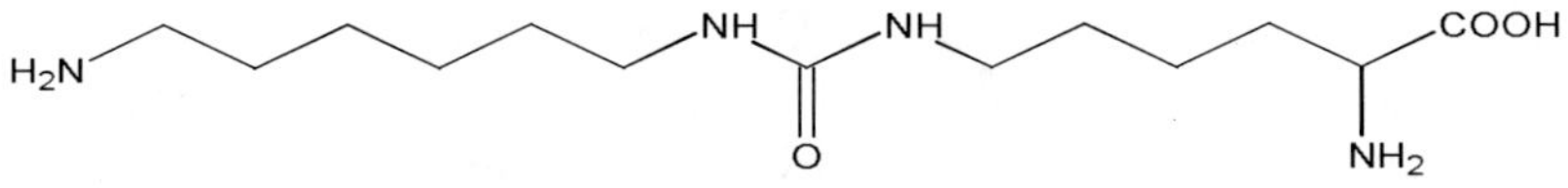

HDI-Lys, FW: 288.4

Figure 5.5. Molecular structure of HDI-Lysine as a biomarker for HDI.

Separately, specific urinary metabolites of MDI exposure have not yet been reported in humans, although detection of dilysine-MDI in the urine of MDI-exposed mice has been reported [Wisnewski et al., 2019]. An investigation [Wisnewski et al., 2022] explored the reactivity of glutathione (GSH) with aliphatic polyisocyanates most commonly used in industry today. LC-MS/MS was used to characterise reaction products generated under physiologic conditions and model their chemical structures. It is found that the aliphatic polyisocyanates readily react with GSH to form primary S-linked tris (GSH)-conjugates, a process that may play an important role in response to respiratory tract exposure. A summary of newly developed biomarkers for biological monitoring exposure to isocyanates in the last decade is shown in Table 5.5.

Table 5.5. Summary of newly developed biomarkers for biological monitoring exposure to isocyanates in the last decade

Study	New Biomarkers	Matrix
Sabbiono 2010	Acetylated MDI-lysine and MDI-lysine	Human plasma
Robins 2017	HDI oligomer, HDA isocyanurate	Human urine
Wisnewski 2019	Di-Lysine-MDI	Mice
Wisnewski 2022	Glutathione-HDI polyisocyanates	Water
Nwoko 2022	Acetylated MDI-lysine	Human urine
Sabbiono 2022	HDI-lysine	Human urine

5.6. Applications

5.6.1. Monitoring Exposure to HDI

HDI is predominately used in spray paints within the motor vehicle repair (MVR) industry, see Table 5.6 for a summary of the studies identified. Seven studies were identified as being from the MVR sector, and two of these are from European countries (UK and Netherlands) [Pronk et al., 2006; Jones et al., 2013]. The number of workers in all these studies varies substantially from 45 (Netherlands) to 995 (UK). The Netherlands study [Pronk et al., 2006] observed urinary HDA levels up to 150.2 µg/g creat (146.5 µmol/mol create). Sampling was carried out at multiple time points throughout the day with the highest mean exposure occurring between the early afternoon and evening. Mean exposures for these time points were all ~ 20 µmol/mol create. This is high compared with the UK study results [Jones et al., 2013] where the maximum result was ~ 20 µmol/mol create and to an Australian study of 196 MVR workers which had almost 100% 'none detects' with only three results above the limit of quantification (LOQ) of 0.5 µmol/mol create [Hu et al., 2017]. Also, the Netherlands may be considered high in comparison to the results from the USA [Gaines 2010] that reported post-shift urine samples with HDA levels between < 0.04 and 65.9 µg/L (~< 0.03 – 47.3 µmol/mol create). Other industry sectors have not been so well studied, with only two UK studies added to the list. These were studies at small- and medium-sized enterprises (SEMs) producing PUR elastomer [Cocker et al., 2009] and a survey of SEMs with a variety of uses [Creely et al., 2006]. Results were reported as total isocyanates (HDA + TDA + MDA + IPDA urine levels) and so it was not possible to compare HDI exposure with other studies. There were a low number of detection in the PUR study [Cocker et al., 2009], with 9 of 13 positive sample results being above the UK biological monitoring guidance value of 1 μmol/mol create showing potential for individual exposure in this industry [HSL 2005].

The relatively new results [Hu et al., 2017] will be compared with the previous two representative studies in MVR. The biological monitoring results done in 2006 from another group (The Center for Risk Assessment in the Work Environment) showed that isocyanate was detected in the urine of about 25% of the spray painters [Pronk et al., 2006]. More recently in 2013, 6% of detectable isocyanate concentration was found in Safety and Health Awareness Days (SHADs) program [Jones et al., 2013] by Health & Safety Executive (HSE). The latest study shows 2.6 % of urine results had a detectable concentration of isocyanates. After having compared these three results, it is found that the latest results were lower than the previous studies done by other research groups. Does this comparison indicate that the Australian MVR industry has performed better than other developed countries in the world in terms of protection against isocyanate exposure? The researchers [Hu et al., 2017] believed that the latest study results with a lower detectable concentration of isocyanate were interpreted with caution. As the analytical method has been vigorously ensured by both an internal quality control program and an external quality assurance program, a few worthwhile considerations are addressed by the researchers below.

It is noted that the MVR shops that participated in the survey had a flexible working environment, which means part-time spray painters were employed or full-time painters worked fewer working hours on the spray painting job. It is found that the short initial half-life of HDA means that the urine sample only represents exposure over the past 2–4 hours (Williams et al., 1999). What possibly happened was that part-time sprayers or sprayers working fewer hours may have been exposed but metabolite concentrations were too low and too quickly excreted to show that an exposure had occurred. Although the sampling instructions were given to the employers and sprayers to provide urine samples at the end of a spraying session, there was no guarantee that all sprayers were compliant.

Table 5.6. Summary of HDI exposure studies of the main processes (Modified from Scholten et al., 2020)

Sector	Study populations (Country, no. workers)	Biomonitoring data Expressed as range (median)	Notable correlations/Comments	References
MVR	USA, n = 15	Plasma HDA: 0.012–0.71(0.061[a]) µg/L	Hb and plasma are weakly associated. Air: correlated with cumulative exposure (Hb: r^2 = 0.34, P < 0.05; P: r^2 = 0.37, P < 0.05) 10×higher Hb adducts than plasma due to cumulative exposure and turnover times. Positive association between HDA-Hb adduct concentration and HDI exposure were strongest with cumulative dermal (n = 12, r^2 = 0.32, P = 0.058), cumulative inhalation (n = 12, r^2 = 0.35, P = 0.042), or cumulative air exposure (n = 12, r^2 = 0.34, P = 0.048).	Flack et al., 2011
	USA, n = 46	Plasma HDA: 0.02–0.92 µg/L	Inhalation correlation, r = 0.22, P = 0.026.	Flack et al., 2010
	USA, n = 48	Urine HDA: <0.04–65.9 µg/L (0.1[a])	Dermal and inhalation exposure were found to be significant predictors of urinary biomarker levels.	Gaines et al., 2010
	USA, n = 15	Urine TAHI:<LOD-1.99µg/L (means) [<LOD-0.39µmol/mol cr.]	TAHI reported for the first. Positive correlation between HDI isocyanurate exposure and total urine TAHI concentration (r = 0.14 with creatinine adjustment).	Robbins et al., 2018
	Australia, n = 196	Only 3 above LOQ (0.5µmol/mol cr.)	Positive spray booths are thought to be just as effective as negative because of their high level of non-detects (*External QA participated*).	Hu et al., 2017
	UK, n = 995	Pre-intervention:1.34 (90%) µmol/mol cr. Intervention: 0.60 (90%) µmol/mol cr Post-intervention: 0.68 (90%) µmol/mol cr	Participants were invited to a Safety and Health Awareness Day (SHAD). Samples taken before and after showed lower results after the intervention	Jones et al., 2013
	Netherlands, N = 55	Urine HDA:<2.9-146.5µmol/mol cr.(means)	The highest concentrations of HDA in urine were seen in the afternoon and early evening. Dermal exposure was a predictor of the presence of HDA.	Pronk et al., 2013

Sector	Study populations (Country, no. workers)	Biomonitoring data Expressed as range (median)	Notable correlations/Comments	References
Other	UK, N = 71	Urine HDA: 56 < LOD, 13 > LOD, 9 > Biological Monitoring Guidance Value <0.5–10.1 (1.8) μmol mol−1 cr.	About 25 companies were visited that were involved in the manufacture of PUR products.	Cocker et al., 2009
	UK, n = 67	Urine HDA: results reported as total isocyanates, HDA most commonly detected n = 21	Low airborne concentrations, only 20% above LOQ. Mixing and pouring tasks are seen as a major potential source of exposure. Biased towards good practice	Creely et al., 2006

[a] Geometric mean (rather than median).

The current trend in the industry is to use water-based paints. "Water-based" does not mean "isocyanate-free", just that it is emulsion based and has reduced levels of solvents. The less solvent content in spray paints help reduction of isocyanate evaporation during spray painting. Quite a number of the MVR shops visited in this survey were using water-based paints and a number were using both. The isocyanate fraction is the major component in the hardener in any urethane paint and always has been. Though for decades now, the amount of free monomeric isocyanate has been greatly reduced from 0.5% to 0.1%. This could also explain some of the lower exposures in the urinary isocyanate and solvent metabolite results in this study.

It is found from this study that the completion of sample context form, along with spot urine collection is highly recommended. The isocyanate exposure monitoring work details such as the type of spray area, type of air-fed mask, spray times and durations, type and make of paint, and volume of paint used for each job, will provide crucial information to interpret the biological analysis results. The Safe-Work NSW Road Map is aiming to reduce exposure to hazardous chemicals and materials by 2022, with the next round of isocyanate biological monitoring in NSW Australia to start soon applying what has been found and learned from this study.

This study involved biological monitoring for the isocyanate monomers only; for HDI it is highly likely that the exposures were mostly oligomers/pre-polymers as it is for most two-pack spray paints. This is particularly important with exposure to HDI in two-pack paints used in MVR where free monomeric HDI is much less than 1% and the remainder is polymeric HDI, uretidone, biuret, isocyanurate (Rosenberg et al., 1986a; Fent et al., 2008). Around the world, the majority of regulations only cover the monomer, but both the monomer and the oligomers should be measured, particularly in relation to worker-related illnesses (Bello et al., 2004). More HDI oligomers were detected than HDI monomers in the air sampling studies in the MVR shops (Fent et al., 2009 a and b]. To measure not only the monomer but also oligomers, in the workplace air concentration has become more prevalent after a recently developed sampling device, the ASSET EZ4 NCO, was put on the market a few years ago [Puscasu et al., 2015a and b].

The current biological monitoring of HDI exposure has been limited to the hydrolysis of the product of HDI monomer, HDA and the proportion of a small percentage of HDI monomer in spray painting has been reduced over the years. One method to face the challenge that the proportion of HDI monomer in spray paints has reduced is to lower the detection limit of the analytical method. Another way is to determine the metabolites of HDI oligomers or other biomarkers associated with HDI and/or its oligomers, which are logically believed to be a more realistic exposure assessment with MVR spray painters.

As discussed in the previous section 5.5.5 Criteria for Selection of a Biomarker, three new biomarkers have been developed to meet this demand. One of these biomarkers was TAHI (trisaminohexyl isocyanurate), a specific metabolite to the oligomer HDI isocyanaurate [Robbins et al., 2018]. TAHI was detected in a third of the 111 exposed workers. Most of the data in the retrieved studies from the MVR described exposure to the HDI monomer (due to methods and standards not being available for oligomer exposure detection in urine prior to 2018) even though oligomers make up the bulk of 2-pack spray paints [Rosenberg and Savolainen 1986 a and b; Fent et al., 2008.; Pronk et al., 2006] also demonstrated significantly higher concentrations of HDI oligomers in personal inhalation samples when compared with HDI monomers. The mean values of NCO (isocyanate content) exposure for sprayers were 2.1 $\mu g/m^3$ of NCO from monomer exposure and 116.3 $\mu g/m^3$ of NCO from oligomer exposure.

In 2022, new biomarkers, (tris) GHS-isocyanate adducts as the major reaction product of GHS with most commonly used contemporary polymeric (tri-isocyanate) formulations of hexamethylene diisocyanate (HDI), the isocyanurate and biuret were identified [Wisnewski et al., 2022]. The study shows that industrially-used aliphatic polyisocyanates readily react with GHS to form primarily S-linked (tris) GHS-conjugates, a process that may play an important role in response to respiratory tract exposure.

In the same year, another new biomarker, HDI-Llysine was found after pronate digestion of albumin [Sabbiono and Pugh, 2022]. This new biomarker can be used to determine isocyanate-specific adducts with albumin in workers exposed to HDI.

5.6.2. Monitoring Exposure to TDI

TDI is a volatile diisocyanate used in foam blowing, glues/adhesives, and lacquers, see Table 5.7 for a summary of the studies identified.

Continuous foam production has been the most studied individual process [six papers from different European Union (EU) countries]' although the number of workers per study was generally small (N < 30) (Table 5.7). Maximum observed results ranged from 3.9 μmil/mol create. [Swierczynska-Machura et al., 2015] to 97 μmol/mol create [Geen 2012].

Moulding processes have been studied in larger (n = 18-90) worker populations than for continuous foam production (n = 4-26) but were only reported in two countries: the UK [Cocker 2009, Keen et al., 2012] and Sweden (Sennbro et al., 2004, Tinnerberg et al., 2014]. If mixed processes (which include some moulding companies but results are not reported separately) are included (Littorin et al., 2007, Sakkinen et al., 2011] then three countries are covered (U, Sweden, and Finland) and maximum results for urinary TDA range from ~3.2 [Tinnerberg et al., 2014] to ~110 μmol/mol create [Sennbro et al., 2004]. If the Sennbro study [2004] is excluded, the results are more comparable across studies, with maximum urine TDA kevels of 3.2 [Tinnerberg et al., 2014], > 6.5 [Keen et al., 2012], only 90th percentile reported, 15.5 [Cocker et al., 2009], ~29.3 [Littorin et al., 2007], and 39 [Sakkinen et al., 2011] being reported; all results in μmol/mol create.

There were very few studies looking at other uses of TDI, such as glues, spray adhesives, or heat guns; these were sometimes included in "mixed" studies involving multiple sites but the results were not reported separately.

5.6.3. Monitoring Exposure to MDI

Available studies on MDI (Table 5.8) are mostly from the PUR sector with five papers classified under PUR production/use [Rosenberg et al., 2002, Sennbro et al., 2006, Robert et al., 2007, Cocker et al., 2009, Keen et al., 2012]. Exposures reported in studies from France [Robert et al., 2012] and Sweden [Sennbro et al., 2006] are in reasonable agreement; urine levels of MDA up to 33.7 μg/g create (19.2 μmol/mol create) in the Robert [Robert et al., 2012] study and 78 μg/L 9~32.6 μmol/mol create) in the Sennbro [Sennbro et al., 2006] study. Low levels were reported in the UK PUR elastomer industry with only 6 of 71 workers sampled having detectable exposures (< 0.5-0.7 μmol/mol create) in one study [Cocker et al., 2009] and a reported 90th percentile of 0.5 μmol/mol create in a second study [Keen et al., 2012]. A study conducted in Finland [Rosenberg et al., 2002] examined exposure to thermal degradation products of PURs in a number of processes including grinding and welding in MVR, milling and turning of PUR-coated metal cylinders, injection moulding, welding, and cutting heating pipes, joint welding, and heat-flexing of PUR floor covering.

Table 5.7. Summary of TDI exposure studies of the main processes (Modified from Scholten et al., 2020)

Sector	Study populations (Country, no. workers)	Biomonitoring data Expressed as range median	Comments	References
Continuous foam production	Poland n = 20	Sum-TDA (U) = <0.01–3.9 µmol/mol cr.	Positive for the geometric mean (GM) in each group (r 0.9) U tot TDA (µmol/mol) = 0.10777_TDI (µg/m³) + 0.2178 [5 ppb TDI = 4.1 µmol/mol cr.] RPE was used and observed to impact TDA(U) results (no correlation between individual urinary TDA concentrations and TDI air concentrations).	Swierczynska-Machura et al., 2015
	UK n = 26, 13 handlers, 13 non	Sum-TDA (U) = <–0.4 to 7 (2.21) µmol/mol cr. (handlers)	No correlation between post-shift urinary TDA concentration and airborne TDI concentrations (r = 0.027). Dermal is considered a significant factor—urine 20× higher for the same airborne exposure.	Austin et al., 2007
	Belgium[a] n = 9	Sum-TDA (U) = 4.4–142.6 (18.01b) µg/l [21 samples] [~3 to ~97 (~12.3) µmol/mol cr.]	TDA (µg/g) = 0.547_TDI (µgm³)–1.636, r = 0.917 [5 ppb TDI =19.2 µg/g, 17.8 µmol/mol cr.] Proposed measuring 'increase over shift' to exclude accumulation (*External QA participated*)	Geens et al., 2012
	Finland n = 17	Sum-TDA (U) = <0.05 to 39 µmol/mol cr.	Good correlation between airborne TDI and urinary TDA in post-shift samples (r = 0.91 and 0.86 for the two different factories studied).	Kaaria et al., 2001
	Sweden n = 6	2,4-TDA(U)/2,6-TDA(U) 0.5–5.4/0.2–4.7 µg/l [~0.3–3.7/0.14–3.2 µmol/mol cr.] 2,4-TDA(P)/2,6-TDA(P) 0.1–14/0.7–12 µg/l	Samples were taken Monday morning so results are not comparable to other studies. Only reported levels 'above reference value'.	Tinnerberg et al., 2014
	Finland n = 17	Sum-TDA(U) 0.2–39(4.9) µmol/mol cr. Sum-TDA(P) 0.4–70.8 (5.6) µg/l Sum_TDA(Hb) 0.012–0.33 (0.047) (nmol/g) (90%) µmol/mol cr. Intervention: 0.60 (90%) µmol/mol cr Post-intervention: 0.68 (90%) µmol/mol cr	Air TDI and plasma TDA correlated (r = 0.91). Plasma and urine TDA well correlated (r = 0.97).	Sakkinen et al., 2011

Table 5.7. (Continued).

Sector	Study populations (Country, no. workers)	Biomonitoring data Expressed as range median	Comments	References
	UK n = 71	Sum-TDA(U) <0.5–15.5 (1.3) µmol/mol cr. 2,6-TDA(U) <0.5–13.2 (0.8) µmol/mol cr. 2,4-TDA (U) <0.5–5.6 (0.7) µmol/mol cr.	The companies visited were involved in the manufacture of PUR products.	Cocker et al., 2009
	UK n = 90	Sum-TDA(U) (µmol/mol cr.) <0.4–6.5 (90% median <LOD)	A positive association was observed in 4 pairs of samples (air and urine). Air levels <LOD at 2/5 sites and only 1/11 samples >WEL (20 µg m^3 NCO)— no further data. 446 samples analysed of which 280 were below the detection limit. A follow-up to Cocker et al. (2009).	Keen et al., 2012
Mixed	Sweden n = 136 (including: moulding, continuous foam-, and flame-lamination plants)	2,6-TDA(U) <0.05–43.1 µg/l [<0.03–29.3 µmol/mol cr.] 2,6-TDA(P) <0.05–62.1 µg/l	Correlation (r > 0.86) with air levels for both urine and plasma for same-day samples. Same sites as Sennbro et al. (2004).	Littorin et al., 2007
	Sweden n = 81	2,4-TDA(U)/2,6-TDA(U)/Sum-TDA(U) <0.1–47 (4.5)/<0.1–115 (3.7)/<0.1–162 (9.7) µg/l [<0.07–32 (3.1)/ –78 (2.5)/–110 (6.6) mmol/mol cr.] 2,4-TDA(P)/2,6-TDA(P)/Sum-TDA(P) <0.1–31 (7.4)/<0.1–42 (6.1)/<0.1–70 (14) µg/l	High correlations between air exposure and urinary biomarker levels (ranging from 0.75 to 0.88) or plasma biomarker levels (ranging from 0.50 to 0.78). 2,6-TDA(U) (µg/l) = 2.7 TDI (ppb) + 0.02 (r = 0.88) [5 ppb = 97 µg/l, ~66 µmol/mol cr.]	Sennbro et al., 2004
	Japan[a] n = 18 (spraying urethane paints)	Individual results not reported except graphically, 2,6-TDA(U) <19 µmol/mol cr.	2,6-TDA(U) (µg/g) = 6.6_TDI (ppb) –1.43 (r = 0.91) [5 ppb = 29 µmol/mol cr.]	Sakai et al., 2005
	Finland[a] n = 6 car repair; n = 15 other PUR processes)	Car Repair Sum-TDA(U) <0.02–0.76 (0.23) µmol/mol cr. Other processes <0.02–0.17 (0.07) µmol/mol cr.	Other processes included milling and turning of PUR-coated metal cylinders, injection moulding of thermoplastic PUR, welding of district heating pipes and joint welding of PUR floor covering.	Rosenberg et al., 2002

[a] Geometric mean rather than the median.

Table 5.8. Summary of MDI exposure studies of the main processes (Modified from Scholten et al., 2020)

Sector	Study populations (Country, no. workers)	Biomonitoring data Expressed as range (median)	Notable corrections/Comments	References
(Rigid) foam production	Finland, n = 57	Urine: 0.015–1.4 (0.13) µmol/mol cr. Plasma: 1.8–2.6 µg/l	Airborne levels (very low or not detected) and task time not associated with urinary biomarker levels.	Säkkinen et al., 2011
	Sweden, n = 18	Urine: 0.5–8.4 µg/l [~0.2–3.5 µmol/mol cr.]	Plasma and urinary MDA correlated after 2 days of no exposure (P > 0.986).	Timmerberg et al., 2014
PUR industry (generic)	France, n = 169 (19 factories)	Urine: <0.1–23.6 µg/l [<0.5–19.25 Mmol/mol cr.]	Association with skin exposure. Elevated pre-shift levels but not cumulative. Higher MDI % in formulations is not associated with higher results.	Robert et al., 2007
	Sweden, n = 18	Urine: 0.3–78 (2) µg/l [~0.13–32.7 (0.8) µmol/mol cr.]	Weak but significant correlations with air. P < 0.01 (U), P < 0.05 (P)	Sennbro et al., 2006
	UK, n = 71	Urine: <0.5–0.7 µmol/mol cr. (only 6+ve/71 results above LoD)	Low levels of isocyanate exposure in the PUR elastomer industry.	Cocker et al., 2009
	UK, n = 90	Urine: 56/326 > LoD, 90% 0.5 µmol/mol cr. (median <LOD)		Keen et al., 2012
	Finland, n = 21	Urine: <0.01–3.1 µmol/mol cr.	Low exposures but he highest levels are seen in pipe layers.	Rosenberg et al., 2002
PUR industry (glue)	Sweden, n = 150	Urine: <LoD–1.8 µg/l [<LoD–0.8 µmol/mol cr.] <LoD–9.4 (heat) µg/l	Higher exposure levels when using heated glue (*External QA participated*).	Littorin et al., 2000
Construction	Switzerland[a], n = 65	Urine: MDA 0.003–3.2 µg/l [~0.001–1.3 µmol/mol cr.] Median (P90) Hb-MDA: 0 (0.177) pmol/g Hb Hb-AcMDA: 2 positive, 2.3 and 3.7 pmol/g Hb	U-MDA-tot correlates with U-AcMDA and Hb-MDA with r = 0.86 and r = 0.39, respectively (P < 0.01). U-AcMDA correlates with Hb-MDA with r = 0.47, (P < 0.01). U-MDA correlates with Hb-MDA (r = 0.38, P = 0.05).	Sabbioni et al., 2007

Table 5.8. (Continued)

Sector	Study populations (Country, no. workers)	Biomonitoring data Expressed as range (median)	Notable corrections/Comments	References
	Switzerland[a], n = 65	Albumin: MDI-Lys 0–899.4 fmol m/g AcMDI-Lys: 0–51.2 fmol m/g	Correlation MDI-Lys with MDA-Hb, r = 0.295 ($P < 0.05$) Same workers as Sabbioni et al., 2007 MDI-Lys levels were compared in a subgroup of construction workers (n = 19) which were analysed prior to isocyanate exposure and after 4–7 months of isocyanate exposure; the MDI-Lys levels increased significantly (Wilcoxon sign test, $P < 0.01$).	Sabbioni et al., 2010
	Finland, n = 21	Urine: <0.1–0.2 μmol/mol cr. Dermal: 88% <2 μg MDI 10 cm^2 on hand	The effect of RPE lowering exposure was seen in post-shift samples but not evening and following morning samples indicating 2 routes of exposure, dermal and inhalation.	Henriks-Eckerman et al., 2015
Other	Switzerland[a], n = 27 (chemical industry)	Urine: MDA 0–10.2 (1.7) nmol/l [–0–0.9 (0.142) μmol/mol cr.] Albumin: MDI-Lys 0–138 pmol/g AcMDI-Lys: 25.6 pmol/g (1 +ve)	Correlation MDI-Lys with MDA-Hb, r = 0.382 ($P < 0.05$).	Sabbioni et al., 2010
	Switzerland, n = 73 (urethane mould production)	Albumin: MDI-Lys = 191 pmol/g (mean) (based on 4 workers with asthma who reported that their last activity with MDI was >3 months ago) MDI-Lys = 750 pmol/g (mean) (n = 5)	Workers with confirmed asthma had significantly higher adduct levels than healthy worker.	Sabbioni et al., 2017
	Germany[a], n = 25	Urine: <500–124 490 pmol/g creatinine [0.004–1.1 μmol/mol cr.] Hb: MDA <0.35–1.12 pmol/g ABP-Val-Hyd 0.15–16.2 pmol/g	No exposure assessment; measurement of Hb adducts and ABP-Val-Hyd reflect long term exposure (up to 120 days)	Gries and Leng, 2013

[a] Country of origin assumed from authors' affiliation, not specifically stated in the paper.

Exposures were low overall (0.01-3.1 μmol/mol create) with pipe layers receiving the highest exposures.

Three papers were identified from the construction industry [Sabbioni et al., 2007, 2010, Henriks-Eckerman et al., 2015]. Urine MDA levels were low for both study groups: 0.017-16.4 nmol/L (~0.001-1.4 μmol/mol create) in a Finnish study [Henriks-Eckerman et al., 2015]. Workers were reported to be involved in a range of activities, including spray foaming which could generate higher exposures, but PPE was used in the majority of cases.

In 2017, Wisnewski explored possible urine biomarkers of MDI exposure in mice after respiratory tract exposure to MDI, such as glutathione (GHS) reaction products (MDI-GHS), and after skin exposure to MDI dissolved in acetone [Wisnewski et al., 2019]. The urinary biomarkers of MDI exposure in mice were identified by research data.

In 2022, a study demonstrated for the first time the detection of acetyl-MDI-lysine conjugates in urine from potentially exposed workers [Nwoko et al., 2022]. Previous studies have reported acetyl-MDI-lysine conjugates in plasma samples [Sabbioni et al., 2007, 2010, 2017] or not in human samples [Wisnewski et al., 2019].

5.7. Conclusion

Biological monitoring is an important tool for protecting workers' health and for controlling exposures to isocyanates. Biological monitoring can have a high relevance and broad application for isocyanates and related occupational exposure scenarios. It needs to be applied in accordance with current ethical standards, respecting the individual rights and freedoms of the workers. Despite this, biological monitoring exposure to isocyanates was still considered a largely underused exposure assessment tool in the occupational safety and health context. The commonly used isocyanates in the workplace partially have a skin notation and likely a dermal uptake and have only an Occupational Exposure Limit (OEL) available. Therefore the health-risk assessment is limited to inhalation risks and is mostly ignoring dermal and oral exposure pathways.

Developments in analytical chemistry are notable towards the analysis of a different class of compounds with one method (multi-method) since highly sensitive instruments can detect a variety of compounds in the same analytical run. This offers possibilities, in the long term, of combining chemical analyses of different types of biomarkers in complex biological monitoring programs, possibly making the analysis of a long list of compounds less costly and more manageable. Further, multi-methods require generic sample preparation procedures that do not compromise sensitivity, precision and accuracy.

In order to ensure high analytical quality and to engage more analytical laboratories in biological monitoring studies on isocyanates, a proficiency testing list for isocyanate metabolites needs to be extended to isocyanate oligomer metabolites.

The issues in biological monitoring exposure to isocyanates in the workplace are still emerging. First, more attention should be paid to the development of health-based biomarkers of exposure based on the dose-effect and dose-response relations. More specific biomarkers need to assess exposure to isocyanates by biological monitoring. Second, there should be a greater focus on the control of dermal exposure at the workplace. Biological monitoring will be a critical tool to address these evolving issues.

Development of more specific biomarkers (U-TAHI for HDI-isocyanurate, HDI-lysine for HDI, MDI-lysine for MDI, etc.) was reported. These are yet to be used widely and there are potential issues with standards (they are not commercially available yet) so demonstrating comparability of results will be difficult initially.

The application of biological monitoring exposure to isocyanates in the workplace has the ultimate goal of better-managing exposure and reducing the occurrence of isocyanate-induced asthma.

One of the examples to achieve the above goal is given below. Currently, there is no proposed limit and uncertainty about the correlation between inhalation exposure and urinary metabolite levels. The European Human Biomonitoring project (HBM4EU) has proposed a study protocol designed in 2022 to assess occupational exposure to isocyanates in five European countries [Jones et al., 2022]. The study will collect urine samples (analysed for isocyanate-derived diamines and acetyl-MDI-lysine), blood samples (analysed for isocyanate-specific IgE and IgG antibodies), etc. In addition, occupational hygiene measurements (air monitoring and skin wipe samples) and questionnaire data will be collected.

The future perspectives with respect to the wider application of biological monitoring exposure to isocyanates in occupational settings and its benefits are [OECD 2022]:

- Facilitate the further implementation of biological monitoring in national Occupational Safety and Health regulations.

- Develop analytical methods for increasing the cost-effectiveness of biological monitoring, without compromising the health protection of workers.
- Consider data-sharing and re-use of biological monitoring data.
- Facilitate the interdisciplinary collaboration between Occupational Safety or Hygiene professionals (more expertise will improve the efficiency and relevance of biological monitoring campaigns).
- Give more attention to the communication of biological monitoring results to the companies (employer & workers), national authorities, scientific communities and the public.
- Assure through regulation that biological monitoring is based on sound scientific and ethical guidelines and solely aimed at better protection of workers' health. This implies risk assessment and management approaches leading to improving the workplaces rather than excluding the more vulnerable workers. Give additional attention to protecting vulnerable populations at work with adequate health and biological monitoring assessments.
- Create a regulatory usable infrastructure allowing a better biological monitoring data exchange between national and international authorities.

References

ACGIH. (2022) *Threshold Limit Values (TLVs) and Biological Exposure Indices* (BEIs). Cincinnati, OH, USA: Signature Publishers.

Adam N, Avar G, Blankenheim H, Friederichs W, Giersig M, Weigand E, Halfmann M, and Wittbecker FW (2005) *Polyurethanes*. In Ullmann's Encyclopedia of Industrial Chemistry. Hoboken, NJ: Wiley-VCH

Allport DC, Gilbert DS, Outterside SM. (2003) *MDI and TDI: safety, health and the environment: a source book and practical guide*. Chichester, UK: John Wiley & Sons.

Aubin S, Hamdi EM, Joly A, Sarazin P, Lesage J, Breau L, Spence M, and Gagné S (2020a) On site comparison of the OSHA 42, Asset EZ4-NCO, Iso-Chek, DAN and CIP10 methods for measuring toluene diisocyanate (TDI) at a polyurethane foam factory. *J Occup Environ Hyg*; **17**: 207-219.

Aubin S, Hamdi EM, Joly A, Sarazin P, Lesage J, Breau L, Spence M, and Gagné S (2020b) On-site comparison of the OSHA 47, Asset EZ4-NCO, Iso-Chek, DAN, and CIP10 methods for measuring methylene diphenyl diisocyanate (MDI) at an oriented-strand board (OSB) factory, *J Occup Environ Hyg;* **17**: 560-573.

Austin S (2007) Biological monitoring of TDI-derived amines in polyurethane foam production. *Occup Med (Lon)*; **57**: 444–448.

Badham C and Taylor HB (1927) 'Lead Poisoning: Concerning the Standards Which Should be Used in Diagnosing this Industrial Disease, Together with a New Method for the Determination of Lead in Urine', *Studies in Industrial Hygiene,* no. 7, Joint Volumes of Papers Presented to the Legislative Council and Legislative Assembly, New South Wales, vol. 1, 1st Session of the 28th Parliament, p. 52.

Bagon DA, Warwick CJ and Brown R (1984), *Am Ind Hyg Assoc J*; **45**: 39.

Baker GB, Coutts RT, Holt A (1994). Derivatization with acetic anhydride: applications to the analysis of biogenic amines and psychiatric drugs by gas chromatography and mass spectrometry. *J Pharmacol Toxicol Methods*; **31**:141–8.

Bayer Corporate Industrial Hygiene Laboratory, *Determination of isocyanates in spray mist environments by sampling with an impinger containing N-(4-nitrobenzyl)-propylamine in toluene and analysis by high performance liquid chromatography,* Bayer, Pittsburgh, PA, 1996, Method No. CIHL 1.4.4.

Bello D, Streicher RP and Woskie SR (2002) Evaluation of the NIOSH draft method 5525 for determination of the total reactive isocyanate group (TRIG) for aliphatic isocyanates in autobody repair shops. *J Environ Monit*; **4**: 351–360.

Bello D, Woskie SR, Streicher RP, Liu Y, Stowe MH, Ellen Eisen A, Ellenbecker MJ, Sparer J, Youngs F, Cullen MR, and Redlich CA (2004) Polyisocyanates in occupational environments: a critical review of exposure limits and metrics. *Am J Ind Med*; **46**: 480–91.

Bello D, Smith TJ, Woski SR, Streicher RP, Boeniger MF, Redlich CA, and Liu Y (2006) An FTIR investigation of isocyanates absorption using in vitro guinea pig skin. *J Environ Monit*; **8**: 523–529.

References

Bello A, Xue Y, Gore R, Woskie S, and Bello D (2019) Assessment and control of exposures to polymeric methylene diphenyl diisocyanate (pMDI) in spray polyurethane foam applicators. *Int J Hyg Environ Health*; **222**: 804–15.

Bello A, Xue Y, Gore R, Woskie S, and Bello D (2020) Exposures and urinary biomonitoring of aliphatic isocyanates in construction metal structure coating. *Int J Hyg Environ Health*; **226**: 113495.

Bennett SB (2017) *Isocyanates: Advances in Research and Applications*, New York, Nova Science Publishers, ISBN: 978-1-53610-875-0.

Bengtström L, Salden M and Stec AA (2016) The role of isocyanates in fire toxicity. *Fire Science Reviews*; **5**: 4-27.

Bernstein IL (1982) Isocyanate-induced pulmonary diseases: a current perpective. *J Allergy Clin Immunol*; **70**: 24-31.

Bhandari D, Ruhl J, Murphy A, McGahee E, Chambers D, and Blount BC (2016) Isotope Dilution UPLC-APCI-MS/MS Method for the Quantitative Measurement of Aromatic Diamines in Human Urine: Biomarkers of Diisocyanate Exposure. *Anal Chem*; **88**: 10687-10692.

Bhandari D, Bowman BA, Patel AB, Chambers DM, De Jesús VR, and Blount BC (2018) UPLC-ESI-MS/MS method for the quantitative measurement of aliphatic diamines, trimethylamine N-oxide, and β-methylamino-l-alanine in human urine. *J Chromatogr B Analyt Technol Biomed Life Sci*; **1083**: 86-92.

Brzeźnicki S and Bonczarowska M (2015) Occupational exposure to selected isocyanates in Polish industry. *Med Pr*; **66**: 291–301.

Brorson T, Skarping G and Nielsen J (1990) Biological monitoring of isocyanates and related amines II. Test chamber exposure of humans to 1,6-hexamethylene-diisocyanate (HDI). *Int Arch Occup Environ Health*; **62**: 385–389.

Brorson T, Skarping G and Sango C (1991) Biological monitoring of isocyanates and related amines IV. 2,4 and 2,6 toluenediamine in hydrolysed plasma and urine after test chamber exposure of humans to 2,4 and 2,6 toluene diisocyanate. *Int Arch Occup Environ Health*; **63**: 253–259.

BS EN ISO/IEC 17025:2005, *General requirements for the competence of testing and calibration laboratories.*

Carbonnelle P, Boukortt S, Lison D, and Buchet JP (1996) Determination of toluenediamines in urine of workers occupationally exposed to isocyanates by high-performance liquid chromatography. *Analyst*; **121**: 663–669.

Carlton GN and England EC (2000) Exposures to 1,6-hexamethylene diisocyanate during polyurethane spray painting in the U.S. Air Force. *J Occup Environ Hyg*; **15**: 705-712.

Ceballos D, Whittaker S, Yost M, Dills RL, Bello D, Thomasen JM, Nylander-French LA, Reeb-Whitaker CK, Peters PM, Weiland EV, and Suydam WW (2011) A Laboratory Comparison of Analytical Methods Used for Isocyanates. *Anal Methods*; **3**: 2478-2487.

Christian Six and Frank Richter (2005) *Isocyanates, Organic*. Ullmann's Encyclopedia of Industrial Chemistry. Weinheim: Wiley-VCH.

Cocker J (2007) Biological monitoring for isocyanates. *Occup Med*; **57**: 391–396.

Cocker J (2011) Biological Monitoring for Isocyanates. *Ann Occup Hyg*; **55**: 127-131.

Cocker J, Cain J, Baldwin P, McNally K, and Jones K (2009) A survey of occupational exposure to 4,4'-methylene-bis (2-chloroaniline) (MbOCA) in the UK. *Ann Occup Hyg*; **53**: 499–507.

Cocker J, Jones K, Leng G, Gries W, Budnik LT, Muller J, Goen T, and Hartwig A. MAK Commission, 2017. Hexamethylene diisocyanate, 2,4-toluene diisocyanate, 2,6-toluene diisocyanate, isophorone diisocyanate and 4,4' -methylene diphenyl diisocyanate – Determination of hexamethylenediamine, 2,4-toluenediamine, 2,6-toluenediamine, isophoronediamine and 4,4' -methylenedianiline in urine using gas chromatography-mass spectrometry [*Biomonitoring Methods,* 2017]. The MAKCollection for Occupational Health and Safety 2017, Vol 2, No 3, 1436–1456.

Cocker J and Jones K (2017) Biological monitoring without limits. *Ann Occup Hyg*; **61**: 401–405.

Commission for the Investigation of Health Hazards of Chemical Compounds in the Work Area. *List of MAK and BAT Values 2007*: Maximum Concentrations and Biological Tolerance Values at the Workplace. Report 43. Wiley-Vch; 2007.

Cook W. Occupational Exposure Levels Worldwide 1987. American Industrial Hygiene Association, 1987.

Creely KS, Hughson GW, Cocker J, and Jones K (2006) Assessing isocyanate exposure in polyurethane industry sectors using biological and air monitoring methods. *Ann Occup Hyg*; **50**: 609–621.

Crespo J and Galán J (1999) Exposure to MDI during the process of insulating buildings with sprayed polyurethane foam. *Ann Occup Hyg*; **43**: 415–9.

Cuno E, Brandt B, Assenmacher-Maiworm H, Buchwald KE, Hahn JU, and Hensel T (2015) *Emissionsverhalten von reaktiven PolyurethanSchmelzkleb stoffen/Emission behavior of reactive polyurethane hot melt adhesives.* Gefahrst Reinhalt Luft; 11–2: 457–64.

Dalene M, Skarping G and Tinnerberg H (1994a) Biological monitoring of hexamethylene diisocyanate by determination of 1,6 hexamethylene diamine as the trifluoroethyl chloroformate derivative using capillary gas chromatography with thermionic and selective-ion detection. *J Chromatogr B Biomed Appl*; **656**: 319–328.

Dalene M, Skarping G and Tinnerberg H (1994b) Thermospray mass spectrometry of aliphatic diamines derivatised with trifluoroethyl chloroformate, with special reference to the biological monitoring of hexamethylenediisocyanate (HDI) and isophoronediisocyanate (IPDI). *Chromatographia*; **38**: 776–780.

Dao A and Bernstein D (2018) Occupational exposure and asthma. *Ann Allergy Asthma Immunol*; **120**: 468-475.

DFG (2022). Deutsche Forschungsgemeinschaft (German Research Foundation). *List of MAK and BAT Values*. Weinheim, Germany: WileyVCH Verlag GmbH.

Dulux Safety Data Sheet (2021a). Product Name: 976-H0111 Luxathene HPX Standard Part B, Reference No: DLXGHSEN00040 Issued: 24 March 2021 Version 4 – see https://www.duluxprotectivecoatings.com.au/products/ranges/luxathane/luxathane-hpx/.

References

Dulux Safety Data Sheet (2021b). Product Name: 976-50357 Durethane Part B Reference No: DLXGHSEN000696 Issued: 12 April 2021 Version: 7.0 – see https://www.duluxprotectivecoatings.com.au/products/ranges/durethane/durethane/

EC 2018, Vincentz Network GmbH & Co. KG. *"Proposed restriction of diisocyanates"*. European Coatings. Retrieved 2018-11-22.

ECHA 2018, *"Restriction proposal on diisocyanates and several authorisation applications agreed by RAC and SEAC"*. echa.europa.eu. ECHA. Retrieved 2018-11-22.

EU Commission, 2020. ECHA, *Joint Task Force ECHA Committee for Risk Assessment (RAC) and Scientific Committee on Occupational Exposure Limits (SCOEL) on Scientific aspects and methodologies related to the exposure of chemicals at the workplace.*

EH40/2005 Workplace exposure limits. *Environmental Hygiene Guidance Note* EH40/2005. HSE Books; 2005. ISBN 0 7176 2977 5.

El-Zaemey S, Glass D, Fritschi L, Darcey E, Carey R, Driscoll T, Abramson M, Si S, Benke G, and Reid A (2018) Isocyanates in Australia: Current exposure to an old hazard, *J Occup Environ Hyg*; **15**: 527-530.

England E, Key-Schwartz R, Lesage J, Carlton G, Streicher R, and Song R (2000a) Comparison of sampling methods for monomer and polyisocyanates of 1,6 hexamethylene diisocyanate during spray finishing operations. *J Occup Environ Hyg*; **15**: 472-478.

England E, Key-Schwartz R, Lesage J, Carlton G, Streicher R, and Song R (2000b). Erratum to: Comparison of sampling methods for monomer and polyisocyanates of 1,6-hexamethylene diisocyanate during spray finishing operations. *J Occup Environ Hyg*; **16**: 1-1.

Falcke H, Holbrook S, Clenahan I, Carretero AL, Sanalan T, Brinkmann T, Roth J, Zerger B, Roudier S, Luis, and Sancho LD (2017) Toluene diisocyanate and methylene diphenyl diisocyanate. In *Best available techniques (BAT) reference document for the production of large volume organic chemicals*. Luxembourg: Publications Office of the European Union.

Fent KW, Jayaraj K, Ball LM, and Nylander-French LA (2008) Quantitative monitoring of dermal and inhalation exposure to 1,6-hexamethylene diisocyanate monomer and oligomers. *J Environ Monit*; **10**: 500–507.

Fent KW, Gaines LG, Thomasen JM, Flack SL, Ding K, Herring AH, Whittaker SG, and Nylander-French LA (2009a) Quantification and statistical modelling part I: breathing-zone concentrations of monomeric and polymeric 1,6-hexamethylene diisocyanate. *Ann Occup Hyg*; **53**: 677–689.

Fent KW, Gaines LGT, Thomasen JM, Flack SL, Ding K, Herring AH, Whittaker SG, and Nylander-French LA (2009b) Quantification and statistical modelling—part II: dermal concentrations of monomeric and polymeric 1,6 hexamethylene diisocyanate. *Ann Occup Hyg*; **53**: 691–702.

Flack SL, Fent KW, Linda G. Gaines T, Thomasen JM, Steve Whittaker S, Ball LM, and ylander-French LA (2010) Quantitative plasma biomarker analysisin HDI exposure assessment. *Ann Occ Hyg*; **54**: 41–54.

Gaines LGT, Fent KW, Flack SL, Thomasen JM, Ball LM, Richardson DB, Ding K, Whittaker SG, Nylander-French LA (2010) Urine 1,6 hexamethylene diamine (HDA) levels among workers exposed to 1,6 hexamethylene diisocyanate (HDI). *Ann Occup Hyg*; **54**: 678–691.

Gannon PFG, Berg AS, Gayosso R, Henderson B, Sax SE, and Willems HMJ (2005) Occupational asthma prevention and management in industry - an example of a global programme. *Occup Med*; **55**: 600-605.

Geens T, Dugardin S, Schockaert A, Cooman GD, and Sprundel MV (2012) Air exposure assessment of TDI and biological monitoring of TDA in urine in workers in polyurethane foam industry. *Occup Environ Med*; **69**: 93–98.

Guglya EB (2000) Determination of isocyanates in air. *J Anal Chem*; **55**: 508–529.

Gui W, Wisnewski AV, Neamtiu I, Gurzau E, Sparer JA, Stowe MH, Liu J, Slade MD, Rusu OA, and Redlich CA (2014) Inception cohort study of workers exposed to toluene diisocyanate at a polyurethane foam factory: initial one-year follow-up. *Am J Ind Med*; **57**: 1207–15.

Gylestam D, Riddar JB, Karlsson D, Dahlin J, Dalene M, and Skarping G (2014) Dry Sampling of Gas-Phase Isocyanates and Isocyanate Aerosols from Thermal Degradation of Polyurethane, *Ann Occup Hyg*; **58**, 28–49.

HCOTN 2018, Health Council of the Netherlands (HCOTN) (2018*). Di and Triisocyanates. Health-based recommendation on occupational exposure limits.* The Hague: Health Council of the Netherlands; publication no. 2018/20 – see https://www.healthcouncil.nl/latest/news/2018/11/28/recommendation-on-occupational-exposure-limit-isocyanates.

Henriks-Eckerman ML, Välimaa J and Rosenberg C (2000) Determination of airborne methyl isocyanate as dibutylamine or 1-(2-methoxyphenyl)piperazine derivatives by liquid and gas chromatography, *Analyst*; **125**: 1949–1954.

Henriks-Eckerman ML, Mäkelä EA, Laitinen J, Ylinen K, Suuronen K, Vuokko A, and Sauni R (2015) Role of dermal exposure in systemic intake of methylenediphenyl diisocyanate (MDI) among construction and boat building workers. *Toxicol Lett*; **232**: 595–600.

Henneken H, Vogel M, and Karst U (2007) Determination of airborne isocyanates. *Anal. Bioanal. Chem*; **387**: 219–236.

Henneken H (2006) Validation of a diffusive sampling method for airborne low-molecular isocyanates using 4-nitro-7-piperazinobenzo-2-oxa-1,3-diazoleimpregnated filters and liquid chromatography-tandem mass spectrometry. *J Chromatogr A*; **1134**:112–121,

Hettick JM and Siegel PD (2011) Determination of the toluene diisocyanate binding sites on human serum albumin by tandem mass spectrometry. *Anal Biochem*; **414**: 232–238.

Hettick JM and Siegel PD (2012) Comparative analysis of aromatic diisocyanate conjugation to human albumin utilizing multiplexed tandem mass spectrometry. *Int J Mass Spectrom*; **309**: 168–175.

References

Hettick JM, Siegel PD, Green BJ, Liu J, and Wisnewski AV (2012) Vapor conjugation of toluene diisocyanate to specific lysines of human albumin. *Anal Biochem*; **421**: 706–711.

Hon C-Y, CE Peters, KJ Jardine, and Arrandale VA (2016) Historical occupational isocyanate exposure levels in two Canadian provinces. *J Occup Environ Hyg*; 14: 1-8.

HSE 1977. *Biological Monitoring in the Workplace. A guide for its practical application to chemical exposure.* HSE Books. ISBN 0 7176 1279 1.

HSE (Health and Safety Executive). 1999a. EH 40/98, *Occupational exposure limits* 199.8. Sudbury, England: HSE Books.

HSE 2005. *Workplace exposure limits. Environmental Hygiene Guidance Note.* HSE Books. ISBN 0 7176 2977 5.

HSE 2010. *WATCH Committee Biological Monitoring for isocyanates.* Available at http://www.hse.gov.uk/aboutus/hsc/iacs/acts/watch/051005/13.pdf. Accessed 19 December 2010.

HSE MDHS 25 (2014), Health and Safety Laboratory: "Organic Isocyanates In Air." In *Methods for the Determination of Hazardous Substances,* HSE Books (ed.). Sudbury, Suffolk, Health and Safety Laboratory, 2014. p. 16.

HSE 2020. Health and Safety Executive. *EH40/2005 Workplace exposure limits.*

HSL 2005. Health and Safety Laboratory. *Biological monitoring for isocyanates.* In *Analysis of urine to assess exposure to isocyanates. Guidance for workers, employers, and occupational health professionals.* Buxton, UK: Health Sciences Group, Health and Safety Laboratory. p. 5.

Hu J, O'Donnell GE, Milosavljevic A, and North S (2014) Biological and air monitoring to assess exposure to isocyanates in motor vehicle repair. *J Health Safety Environ*; **30**: 103–112.

Hu J (2016) The role of biological monitoring in assessment of isocyanate exposure in workplaces. *J Health Safety Environ*; **32**: 87-100.

Hu J (2017) The roles of biological monitoring and health surveillance in isocyanates exposure in workplaces, in Bennett SG, *Isocyanates: Advances in Research and Applications*. New York, Nova Science Publishers, ISBN: 978-1-53610-875-0.

Hu J, Cantrell P and Nand A (2017) Comprehensive biological monitoring to assess isocyanates and solvents exposure in the NSW Australia motor vehicle repair, *Ann Work Exp Health*; **61**: 1015–1023.

IARC (1999) *Re-evaluation of some organic chemicals, hydrazine and hydrogen peroxide.*

IARC Working Group on the Evaluation of Carcinogenic Risks to Humans (IARC : Lyon, France), *Monograph 71* – see https://monographs.iarc.who.int/monographs-available/.

IARC 71-37, *"Toluene Diisocyanates"* (PDF). Retrieved 2018-11-18.

IARC 71-47, *4,4'-Methylenediphenyl Diisocyanate and Polymeric 4,4'-methylenediphenyl diisocyanate"* (PDF). Retrieved 2018-11-18.

Ibanez M, Sancho JV, Pozo OJ, Lee F, Wu JT, and Qian MG (2005) A novel liquid chromatography/tandem mass spectrometry-based depletion method for measuring red blood cell partitioning of pharmaceutical compounds in drug discovery. *Rapid Commun Mass*; **19**: 169-178.

References

III 2918, *"Welcome to the International Isocyanate Institute"*. Retrieved 2018-11-18.

ISO 16702: *Workplace air quality — Determination of total organic isocyanate groups in air using 1-(2-methoxyphenyl)piperazine and liquid chromatography.*

ISO 17734-1, *Determination of organonitrogen compounds in air using liquid chromatography and mass spectrometry — Part 1: Isocyanates using dibutylamine derivatives.*

ISO 17735, *Workplace atmospheres — Determination of total isocyanate groups in air using the 1-(9-anthracenylmethyl) piperazine (MAP) reagent and liquid chromatography.*

ISO 17736, *Workplace air — Determination of isocyanates in air using a double-filter sampler and analysis by liquid chromatography.*

ISO 17737, *Workplace atmospheres- guidelines for selecting analytical methods for sampling and analyzing isocyanates in air.*

ISO/IEC 17025:2018, *General requirements for the competence of testing and calibration laboratories.*

Jones K, Cocker J and Piney M (2013) Isocyanate exposure control in motor vehicle paint spraying: evidence from biological monitoring. *Ann Occup Hyg*; **57**: 200–209.

Jones K, Johnson PD, Baldwin PE, Coldwell M, Cooke J, Keen C, Harding AH, Smith D, and Cocker J (2017) Exposure to diisocyanates and their corresponding diamines in seven different workplaces. *Ann Work Exp Health*; **61**: 383–393.

Jones K (2019) Biological monitoring for isocyanates. *Occup Med*; **69**: 515-517.

Jones K, Galea GS, Scholten B, Loikala M, Porras SP, Bousoumah R, Ndaw S, Leese E, Louro H, Silva MJ, Viegas S, Godderis L, Verdonck J, Poels K, Göen T, Duca RC, Santonen T, and HBM4EU Diisocyanates Study Team (2022) HBM4EU Diisocyanates Study-Research Protocol for a Collaborative European Human Biological Monitoring Study on Occupational Exposure. *Int J Environ Res Public Health*; **19**: 8811.

Karria K, Hirvonen A, Norppa H, Piirilä P, Vainio PH, and Rosenberg C (2001a) Exposure to 2,4- and 2,6-toluene diisocyanate during production of flexible foam: determination of airborne TDI and urinary 2,4- and 2,6-toluenediamine (TDA). *Analyst*; **126**: 1025–1031.

Karria K, Hirvonen A, Norppa H, Piirilä P, Vainio PH, and Rosenberg C (2001b) Exposure to 4,4'-methylenediphenyl diisocyanate (MDI) during moulding polyurethane foam: determination of airborne MDI and urinary 4,49-methylenedianiline (MDA). *Analyst*; **126**: 476–479.

Keen C, Coldwell M, McNally K, Baldwin McAlinden PJ, and Cocker J (2012) A follow up study of occupational exposure to 4,4'-methylene-bis(2-chloroaniline) (MbOCA) and isocyanates in polyurethane manufacture in the UK. *Toxicol Lett*; **213**: 3–8.

Key-Schwartz RJ and Tucker S (1999) *Am Ind Hyg Assoc J*; **60**: 200-207.

Klaassen, CD. Casarett and Doull's Toxicology: *The Basic Science of Poisons*. Mcgraw-Hill Medical Publishing Division; 2001.

Kreis K, Aumann-Suslin I, Lüdeke A, Wegewitz U, Zeidler J, and Schulenburg JG (2019) Costs of isocyanate-related occupational diseases: A systematic review, *J Occup Environ Hyg*; **16**: 446-466.

References

Kumar A, Dongari N, and Sabbioni G (2009) New Isocyanate-Specific Albumin Adducts of 4, 40-Methylenediphenyl Diisocyanate (MDI) in Rats. *Chem. Res. Toxicol*; **22**: 1975–1983.

Lepine M, Sleno L, Lesage J, and Gagné S (2019) A validated liquid chromatography/tandem mass spectrometry method for 4,4'-methylenedianiline quantitation in human urine as a measure of 4,4'-methylene diphenyl diisocyanate exposure. *Rapid Commun Mass Spectrom*; **33**: 600-606.

Lépine M, Sleno L, Lesage J, and Gagné S (2020) A validated UPLC-MS/MS method for the determination of aliphatic and aromatic isocyanate exposure in human urine. *Anal Bioanal Chem*; **412**:753–762.

Lesage J, Stanley J, Karoly WJ, and Lichtenberg FW (2007) Airborne methylene diphenyl diisocyanate (MDI) concentrations associated with the application of polyurethane spray foam in residential construction. *J Occup Environ Hyg*; **4**:145–155.

Levine SP, Hilling KJD, and Dharmarajan V (1995) Critical review of methods of sampling, analysis, and monitoring for TDI and MDI. *Am Ind Hyg Assoc J*; **56**: 581.

Lewalter J, Gries W, 2000. Examiners: Angerer J, Sabbioni G, Haemoglobin adducts of aromatic amines: aniline, o-, m- and p-toluidine, o-anisidine, pchloroaniline, α-and β-naphthylamine, 4-aminodiphenyl, benzidine, 4,4' -diaminodiphenylmethane, 3,3' -dichlorobenzidine [*Biomonitoring Methods,* 2000]. The MAK-Collection for Occupational Health and Safety: Wiley-VCH Verlag GmbH & Co. KGaA; Vol 7, 191-219.

Li Z, Mayer RJ, Ofial AR, and Mayr H (2020) From Carbodiimides to Carbon Dioxide: Quantification of the Electrophilic Reactivities of Heteroallenes. *J Am Chem Soc*; **142**: 8383–8402.

Liljelind I, Norberg C, Egelrun L, Westberg H, Eriksson K, and Nylander-French LA (2010) Dermal and inhalation exposure to methylene bisphenyl isocyanates (MDI) in iron foundry workers. *Ann Occup Hyg*; **54**: 31–40.

Lind P, Dalene M, Skarping G, and Hagmar L (1996) Toxicokinetics of 2,4 and 2,6 toluene diamine in hydrolysed urine and plasma after occupational exposure or 2,3 and 2,6 toluene diisocyanate. *Occup Environ Med*; **53**: 94–99.

List of MAK and BAT values 2009 *Commission for the investigation of health hazards of chemical compounds in the work area.* Report No 45. Weinheim, Germany: Wiley-VCH Verlag GmbH, 2009.

Littorin M, Axmon A, Broberg K, Sennbro CT, and Tinnerberg H (2007) Eye and airway symptoms in low occupational exposure to toluene diisocyanate. *Scand J Work Environ Health*; **33**: 280–285.

Luna LG, Green BJ, Zhang F, Arnold SM, Siegel PD, and Bartelsa MJ (2014) Quantitation of 4, 4'-methylene diphenyl diisocyanate human serum albumin adducts. *Toxicol Rep*; **1**: 743–751.

Mackie J (2008) Effective health surveillance for occupational asthma in motor vehicle repair. *Occup Med*; **58**: 551–555.

Maitre A, Berode M, Perdix A, Romazini S, and Savolainen H (1993) Biological monitoring of occupational exposure to toluene diisocyanate. *Int Arch Occup Environ Health*; **65**: 97–100.

Maitre A, Berode M, Perdix A, Stoklov M, Mallion JM, and Savolainen H (1996) Urinary hexane diamine as an indicator of occupational exposure to hexamethylenediisocyanate. *Int Arch Occup Environ Health*; **69**: 65–68.

Manini P, De Palma G and Mutti A (2007) Exposure assessment at the workplace: implications of biological variability. *Toxicol Lett*; **168**: 210–218.

Manno M and Viau C (2010) Biomonitoring for occupational health risk assessment. *Toxicol. Lett*; **193**: 3-16.

Marand A, Karlsson D, Dalene M, and Skarping G (2004) Determination of amines as pentafluoropropionic acid anhydride derivatives in biological samples using liquid chromatography and tandem mass spectrometry. *Analyst*; **129**: 522–528.

Marand A, Karlsson D, Dalene M, and Skarping G (2005) Solvent-free sampling with di-n-butylamine for monitoring of isocyanates in air. *J Environ Monit*; **7**: 335–343.

McDonald JC, Chen Y, Zekveld C, Cherry NM (2005) Incidence by occupation and industry of acute work related respiratory diseases in the UK, 1992–2001. *Occup Environ Med*; **62**: 836–842.

MDHS 25/4, Health and Safety Laboratory: Organic Isocyanates in Air. In *Methods for the Determination of Hazardous Substances,* HSE Books (ed.). Sudbury, Suffolk, Health and Safety Laboratory, 2014. p. 16.

Mhike M, Chipinda I, Hettick JM, Simoyi RH, Lemons A, Green BJ, and Siegel PD (2013) Characterization of methylene diphenyl Diisocyanatehaptenated human serum albumin and hemoglobin. *Anal Biochem*; **440**: 197–204.

Miles Corporate Industrial Hygiene Laboratory, *Determination of isocyanates in spray mist environments by sampling in an impinger with N-4-nitrobenzyl-N-n-propylamine in toluene and analysis by high performance liquid chromatography*, Miles, Pittsburgh, PA, 1992, Method 1.4.3.

Morgan MS and Schaller KH (1999) An analysis of criteria for biological limit values developed in Germany and in the United States. *Int Arch Occup Environ Health*; **72**: 195–204.

Mutti A, De Palma G, Manini P (2006). In: SIMLII (Ed.), *Guidelines for biological Monitoring*. Maugeri Foundation Books, Pavia, p.22.

NIOSH (1987). NIOSH Method 2535, *Toluene 2,4-diisocyanate.*

NIOSH (1989). NIOSH Method 5521, *Isocyanates, monomeric.*

NIOSH (1996). NIOSH Method 5522, *Isocyanates.*

NIOSH (2003). NIOSH Method 5525, *Isocyanates,* Total (MAP).

NMCPHC 2018, Medical Surveillance Procedures Manual and Medical Matrix (edition 11) (PDF). Navy and Marine Corps Public Health Center. Retrieved 2018-11-21.

NOHSC 1995. National Occupational Health and Safety Commission. *Guidelines for Health Surveillance.* [NOHSC: 7039(1995)]. Adopted national exposure standards for atmospheric contaminants in the occupational environment. NOHSC: 1003. Available from the Australian Safety and Compensation Council (www.ascc.gov.au).

Nordqvist Y, Nilsson U, Colmsjo A, Dahl A, and Gudmundsson A (2005) A chemosorptive cylindrical denuder designed for personal exposure measurements of isocyanates-evaluation on generated aerosols of 4,4'-methylenediphenyl diisocyanate. *J Environ Monit*; **7**: 469–474.

NTP (National Toxicology Program) (2021) Report on Carcinogens. Fifteenth Edition. Research Triangle Park, NC, USA: U.S. Department of Health and Human Services.

Nwoko KC, Kenny L and Jones K (2022) Methylenediphenyl diisocyanate lysine conjugates in the urine of workers exposed to methylenediphenyl diisocyanate. *Toxicol Ind Health*; **38**: 636–642.

OECD 2022, *Occupational Biomonitoring Guidance Document*, Series on Testing and Assessment No. 370

Omega Specialty Instrument Co. (2006). *ISO-CHEK® Sampling Protocol*. Retrieved 12 2012, from http://www.omegaspec.com/kbase/ShowKbase.asp?Article=203

OSHA 42. Occupational Safety and Health Administration (OSHA), *Diisocyanates:* method 42, U.S. Department of Labor, OSHA, Salt Lake City, UT, 1983.

OSHA (1983). OSHA Method 42, *Diisocyanates*.

OSHA (1984). OSHA Method 47, *Methylene Bisphenyl Isocyanate (MDI)*.

OSHA (2022). OSHA Method 5002, 8 *Isocyanate monomers*.

Pauluhn J and Lewalter J. (2002) Analysis of markers of exposure to polymeric methylenediphenyl diisocyanate (pMDI) in rats: a comparison of dermal and inhalation exposure. *Exp Toxic Pathol*; **53**: 135–146.

Paustenbach DJ: *Occupational Exposure Limits*. In Encyclopaedia Of Occupational Health And Safety. 4th Ed. (Vol. 1), J. M. Stellman (Ed.) Geneva: International Labour Office, 1998. Pp. 30.27–30.34.

Polkowska Z, Kozłowska K, Namiesnik J, and Przyjazny A (2004) Biological fluids as a source of information on the exposure of man to environmental chemical agents. *Crit Rev Anal Chem*; **34**: 105–119.

Pronk A, Tielemans E, Skarping G, Bobeldijk I, Hemmen JV, Heederik D, and Preller L (2006a) Inhalation exposure to isocyanates of car body repair shop workers and industrial spray painters. *Ann Occup Hyg*; **50**: 1–14.

Pronk A, Yu F, Vlaanderen J, Tielemans E, Preller L, Bobeldijk I, Deddens JA, Latza U, Baur X, and Heederik D (2006b) Dermal, inhalation, and internal exposure to 1,6-HDI and its oligomers in car body repair shop workers and industrial spray painters. *Occup Environ Med*; **63**: 624–631.

Puscasu S, Aubin S, Tra HV, and Gagné S (2014) Adaptation of CIP10 for the sampling of 4,4′-methylene diphenyl diisocyanate aerosols, *Anal Methods*; **6**: 1101-1107.

Puscasu S, Aubin S, Y. Cloutier Y, Sarazin P, Tra HV, and Gagné S (2015a) CIP10 optimization for 4,4-methylene diphenyl diisocyanate aerosol sampling and field comparison with impinger method. *Ann Occup Hyg*; **59**: 347–357.

Puscasu S, Aubin S, Cloutier Y, Sarazin P, Tra HV, and Gagné S (2015b) Comparison between the ASSET EZ4 NCO and impinger sampling devices for aerosol sampling of 4,4'-methylene diphenyl diisocyanate in spray foam application. *Ann Occup Hyg*; **59**: 872–81.

Puscasu S, Aubin S, Sarazin P, Richard L, Spence M, and Gagné S (2017) Use of the Novel Derivatizing Agent 1,8-Diaminonapthalene With the CIP10 Sampler to Measure 4,4'-Methylene Diphenyl Diisocyanate Atmospheres, *Ann Work Expo Health*; **61**: 566–574.

Rando RJ, Poovey HG, and Mokadam D R (2001) *Evaluation of the ISOCHEK Sampler for Measurement of Monomers and Prepolymers of TDI and MDI, Project 155, Reference 11415.* International Isocyanate Institute, Inc., Manchester, UK

Rando RJ, Poovey HG and Mokadam D R (2002) *Laboratory comparission of sampling methods for reactive isocyanate vapour and aerosols, Isocyanates: sampling, analysis, and health effects,* ASTM STP 1408, J. Lesage, I.D. DeGraft, and R.S. Danchik, Eds., American Society for Testing and Materials, West Conshohocken, PA.

Redlich CA and Herrick CA (2008) Lung/skin connections in occupational lung disease. *Curr Opin Allergy Clin Immunol*; **8**: 115–119.

Reeb-Whitaker C, Whittaker SG, Ceballos DM, Weiland EC, Sheila L. Flack SL, Fent KW, Thomasen JM, Trelles LGT Gaines, and Nylander-French LA (2012). Airborne isocyanate exposures in the collision repair industry and a comparison to occupational exposure limits. *J Occup Environ Hyg*; **9**: 329-339.

Reinhard R and Ulrich H (1977) "Syntheses and Preparative Applications of Isocyanates". In Saul Patai (ed.). Cyanates and Their Thio Derivatives: Part 2, Volume 2. *PATAI'S Chemistry of Functional Groups.* pp. 619–818. doi:10.1002/9780470771532.ch1. ISBN 9780470771532.

Richter R and Henri U (1977) *Syntheses and Preparative Applications of Isocyanates.* In Saul Patai (ed.). Cyanates and their Thio Derivatives: Part 2, Volume 2. PATAI'S Chemistry of Functional Groups. pp. 619–818. ISBN 9780470771532.

Robbins Z, Bodnar W, Zhang Z, Gold A, and Nylander-French LA (2018) Trisamino-hexyl isocyanurate, a urinary biomarker of HDI isocyanurate exposure. *J Chromatogr B Analyt Technol Biomed Life Sci*; **1076**: 117-129.

Roberge B, Gravel R, Drolet D (2009) *4,4'-Diphenylmethane diisocyanate (MDI)— safety practices and concentration during polyurethane foam spraying.* Montréal, CA: Institut de recherche Robert-Sauvé en santé et en sécurité du travail (IRSST).

Roberge B, Aubin S, Ostiguy C, Lesage J. (2013). *Guide for Safe Use of Isocyanates – An Industrial Hygiene Approach.* Institut de recherche Robert-Sauvé en santé et en sécurité du travail (IRSST) publication RG-773 – see http://www.irsst.qc.ca/media/documents/PubIRSST/RG-773.pdf.

Robert A, Ducos P, Francin JM, and Marsan P (2007) Biological monitoring of workers exposed to 4,4'-methylenediphenyl diisocyanate (MDI) in 19 French polyurethane industries. *Int Arch Occup Environ Health*; **80**: 412–242.

Rosenberg C and Saviolainen H (1986a) Determination in urine of diisocyanate-derived amines from occupational exposure by gas chromatography-mass spectrometry. *Analyst*; **111**: 1069–1071.

Rosenberg C and Saviolainen H (1986b) Determination of occupational exposure to toluene diisocyanate by biological monitoring. *J Chromatogr*; **367**: 385–392.

Rosenberg C, Nikkila K, Henriks-Eckerman M, Peltonen K, and Engströrm K (2002) Biological monitoring of aromatic diisocyanates in workers exposed to thermal degradation products of polyurethanes. *J Environ Monit*; **4**: 711–716.

Rother D & Schlüter U (2021) Occupational exposure to diisocyanates in the European Union. *Ann Work Expo Health*; **65**: 893-907.

Robert W, Wood R, Andersen J (2014) Spray polyurethane foam monitoring and reoccupancy of high pressure open cell applications to new residential constructions. In *Polyurethanes Technical Conference,* Dallas, TX.

Rudzinski WE, Yin J, England E, Key-Schwartz R, and Lesage J (2001) A comparison of solid sampler methods for the determination of hexamethylene-based isocyanates in spray-painting operations. *AIHAJ : A Journal for the Science of Occupational and Environmental Health and Safety,* **62**: 246-250.

Sabbioni G, Beyerbach A. (2000) Haemoglobin adducts of aromatic amines: diamines and polyaromatic amines. *J. Chromatogr. B Biomed. Sci. Appl*; **744**: 377–387.

Sabbioni G, Hartley R, Henschler D, Höllrigl-Rosta A, Koeber R, and Schneider S (2000) Isocyanate-specific hemoglobin adduct in rats exposed to 4, 4'-methylenediphenyl diisocyanate. *Chem. Res. Toxicol*; **13**, 82–89.

Sabbioni G and Beyerbach A (2000) Haemoglobin adducts of aromatic amines: diamines and polyaromatic amines. *J. Chromatogr. B Biomed. Sci. Appl*; **744**: 377–387.

Sabbioni G, Wesp H, Lewalter J, and Rumler R (2007) Determination of isocyanate biomarkers in construction site workers. *Biomarkers*; **12**: 468–483.

Sabbioni G, Dongari N, and Kumar A (2010) Determination of a new biomarker in subjects exposed to 4,4'-methylenediphenyl diisocyanate. *Biomarkers*; **15**: 508–515.

Sabbioni G, Dongari N, Kumar A, and Baur X (2016) Determination of albumin adducts of 4, 40-Methylenediphenyl diisocyanate after specific inhalative challenge tests in workers. *Toxicol Lett*; **260**: 46–51.

Sabbioni G and Turesky RJ (2017) Biomonitoring human albumin adducts: the past, the present, and the future. *Chem. Res. Toxicol.* **30**, 332–366.

Sabbioni G and Pugh SA (2022) New Method to Biomonitor Workers Exposed to 1,6-Hexamethylene Diisocyanate. *Chem. Res. Toxicol*; **35**: 2285–2295.

Safe Work Australia. *Guidance on the Interpretation of Workplace Exposure Standards for Airborne Contaminants*; April 2013. Available from: www.safeworkaustralia.gov.au/sites/swa/about/publications/pages/workplace-exposure-standards-airborne-contaminants.

Safe Work Australia. *Hazardous Substances Information System (HSIS).* Available from: hsis.safeworkaustralia.gov.au/ExposureStandards/Details?exposureStandardID=586.

SafeWork NSW. (2023) *Chemical analysis branch handbook-workplace and biological exposure analysis.* 9th ed. New South Wales, Australia. Available online: https://www. nsw.gov.au/sites/default/files/2022-02/TestSafe-ChemicalAnalysis-Branch-Handbook-9th-edition-TS033.pdf. Accessed on 6 January, 2023.

Sakai T, Morita Y, Kim Y, and Tao YX (2002) LC-MS determination of urinary toluenediamine in workers exposed to toluenediisocyanate. *Toxicol Lett*; **134**: 259–264.

Säkkinen K, Tornaeus J, Hesso A, Hirvonen A, Vainio H, Norppa H, and Rosenberg C (2011) Protein adducts as biomarkers of exposure to aromatic diisocyanates in workers manufacturing polyurethane (PUR) foam. *J Environ Mon*it; **13**: 957–65.

Sandstrom JF, Skarping G and Dalene M (1989) Chromatographic determination of amines in biological fluids with special reference to the biological monitoring of isocyanates and amines: II. Determination of 2,4- and 2,6-toluenediamine using glass capillary gas chromatography and selected ion monitoring. *J Chromatogr A*; **479**: 135-143.

Schupp T and Plehiers PM (2022) Absorption, distribution, metabolism, and excretion of methylene diphenyl diisocyanate and toluene diisocyanate: Many similarities and few differences. *Toxicol Ind Health*; **38**: 500-528.

Schutze D, Sepai O, Lewalter J, Miksche L, Henschler D, and Sabbioni G (1995) Biomonitoring of workers exposed to 4,4' methylenedianiline or 4,4'-methylenediphenyl diisocyanate. *Carcinogensis*; **16**: 573–582.

Sekizawa J and Greenberg MM (2000) *Concise International Chemical Assessment Document 27: Diphenylmethane diisocyanate (MDI)*. Retrieved 2018-11-18.

Semple S (2004) Dermal exposure to chemicals in the workplace: just how important is skin absorption? *Int Arch Occup Environ Health*; **61**: 376–382.

Sennbro CJ, Lindh CH, Tinnerberg H, Gustavsson C, Littorin M, Welinder H, and Jönsson BAG (2003) Development, validation and characterization of an analytical method for the quantification of hydrolysable urinary metabolites and plasma protein adducts of 2,4- and 2,6-toluene diisocyanate, 1,5 naphthalene diisocyanate and 4,4'-methylendiphenyl diisocyanate. *Biomarkers*; **8**: 204–217.

Sennbro CJ, Lindh CH, Tinnerberg H, Welinder H, Littorin M, and Jönsson BAG (2004) Biological monitoring of exposure to toluene diisocyanate. *Scan J Work Environ Health*; **30**: 371–378.

Sennbro CJ, Littorin M, Tinnerberg H, and Jonsson BAG (2005) Upper reference limits for biomarkers of exposure to aromatic diisocyanates. *Int Arch Occup Environ Health*; **78**: 541–546.

Sennbro CJ, Lindh CH, Mattson C, Jönsson BAG, and Tinnerberg H (2006) Biological monitoring of exposure to 1,5-naphthalene diisocyanate and 4,4'-methylenediphenyl diisocyanate. *Int Arch Occup Environ Health*; **79**: 647–653.

Sepai O, Schutze D, Heinrich U, Hoymann HG, Henschler D, and Sabbioni G (1995) Hemoglobin adducts and urine metabolites of 4,49-methylenedianinine after 4,4'-methylenediphenyl diisocyanate exposure of rats. *Chem Biol Interact*; **97**: 185–198.

SFMT (Société Française de Médecine du Travail) (2016)/SFMT (French Society of Occupational Medicine) (2016), *Surveillance biologique des expositions professionnelles aux agents chimiques/Recommendations for good practice. Biological monitoring of occupational exposure to chemical agents*, Recommandations de bonne pratique. Available on request.

Sigma-Aldrich Co. LLC (2013). *ASSET EZ4-NCO Dry Sampler for Isocyanates*. Retrieved January 2014, from Sigma-Aldrich: http://www.sigmaaldrich.com/analytical-chromatography/air-monitoring/asset-ncosampler.Html

Six C and Richter F (2005) "Isocyanates, Organic". Ullmann's Encyclopedia of Industrial Chemistry. Weinheim: Wiley-VCH.

Skarping G, Brorson T and Sango C (1991) Biological monitoring of isocyanates and related amines III. Test chamber exposures of humans to toluene diisocyanate. *Int Arch Occup Environ Health*; **63**: 83–88.

Skarping G, Dalene M and Tinnerberg H (1994) Biological monitoring of hexamethylene and isophorone-diisocyanate by the determination of hexamethylenediamine and isophoronediamine in hydrolysed urine using liquid chromatography and mass spectrometry. *Analyst*; **119**: 2051–2055.

Skarping G and Dalene M (1995) Determination of 4,4'- methylenediphenyldianiline (MDA) and identification of isomers in technical-grade MDA inhydrolysed plasma and urine from workers exposed to methylenediphenyldiisocyanate by gas chromatography-mass spectrometry. *J Chromatogr B Biomed Appl*; **663**: 209–216.

SKC Iso-Chek (2017) https://www.skcltd.com/images/pdfs/ISO-CHEK_1637_Feb_2017.pdf

Skoog DA, Holler FJ, Crouch SR (2017) *Principles of Instrumental Analysis*, Edition 7, Publisher Cengage Learning.

Smolders R, Schramm KW, Nickmilder M, and Schoeters G (2009) Applicability of non-invasively collected matrices for human biomonitoring. *Environ Health*; **8**: 1–10.

Sparer J, Stowe MH, Bello D, Liu Y, Gore RJ, Youngs F, Cullen MR, Redlich CA, and Woskie SR (2004) Isocyanate exposures in autobody shop work: the SPRAY study. *J Occup Environ Hyg*; **1**: 570–581.

Streicher RP, Kennedy ER and Lorberau CD (1994) Strategies for the simultaneous collection of vapours and aerosols with emphasis on isocyanate sampling. *Analyst*; **119**: 89.

Streicher RP, Arnold JE, Ernst MK, and Cooper CV (1996) Development of a novel derivatization reagent for the sampling and analysis of total isocyanate group in air and comparison of its performance with that of several established reagents. *Am Ind Hyg Assoc J*; **57**: 905-913.

Streicher RP, Reh CM, Key-Schwartz RJ, Schlecht PC, Cassinelli ME, and O'Connor PF (2000) Determination of airborne isocyanate exposure: Considerations in method selection. *Am Ind Hyg Assoc J*; **61**:544–556.

Streicher RP, Reh CM, Key-Schwartz RJ, and O'Connor PF (2002) Selecting Isocyanate Sampling and Analytical Methods. *Appl. Occup. Environ. Hyg*; **17**: 157-162.

Supelco Analytical. (2013). *Extraction and Analysis of ASSETTM EZA-NCO Dry Sampler*. Rev 1.5. Bellefonte: Supel.

SWA (2013). Safe Work Australia. *Guidance on the Interpretation of Workplace Exposure Standards for Airborne Contaminants*. Available from: www.safeworkaustralia.gov.au/sites/swa/about/publications/pages/workplace-exposure-standards-airborne-contaminants.

SWA (2015). *Deemed Diseases in Australia*. Prepared for Safe Work Australia by Prof T Driscoll, August 2015 – see https://www.safeworkaustralia.gov.au/doc/deemed-diseases-australia.

SWA (2021). *Hazardous Chemical Information System (HCIS)*. Safe Work Australia website – see http://hcis.safeworkaustralia.gov.au/HazardousChemical.

Swierczynska-Machura D, Brzeznicki S, Nowakowska-Swirta E, Walusiak-Skorupa J, Wittczak T, Dudek W, Bonczarowska M, Wesolowski W, Czerczak S, and Pałczyński C (2015) Occupational exposure to diisocyanates in polyurethane foam factory workers. *Int J Occup Med Environ Health*; **28**: 985-998.

Thomasen JM, Fent KW, Reeb-Whitaker C, Whittaker SG, and Nylander-French LA (2011). Field comparison of air sampling methods for monomeric and polymeric 1,6-hexamethylene diisocyanate. *J Occup Environ Hyg*; **8**: 161-178.

Timchalk KC, Smith FA and Bartels MJ (1994) *Toxical Appl Pharmacol*; **124**:181-190.

Tinnerberg H, Skarping G, Dalene M, and Hagmar L (1995) Test chamber exposure of humans to 1,6-hexamethylene diisocyanate and isophorone diisocyanate. *Int Arch Occup Environ Health*; **67**: 367–374.

Tinnerberg H and Mattsson C (2008) Usage of air monitoring and biomarkers of isocyanates exposure to assess the effect of a control intervention. *Ann Occup Hyg*; **52**: 187–194.

Tinnerberg H, Broberg K, Lindh CH, and Jonsson BAG (2014) Biomarkers of exposure in Monday morning urine samples as a long-term measure of exposure to aromatic diisocyanates. *Int Arch Occup Environ Health*; **87**: 365–72.

Tiljander A, Skarping G and Dalene M (1989) Chromatographic determination of amines in biological fluids with special reference to the biological monitoring of isocyanates and amines III determination of 4'4'methylenedianiline in hydrolysed humanurine using derviatization and capillary gas chromatography with selected ion monitoring. *J Chromatogr*; **479**: 142–152.

TRGS 150: Unmittelbarer Hautkontakt mit Gefahrstoffen. Bundesarbeitsbl. 47, 10/1987.

US EPA 2015, OCSPP, OPPT, EETD (2015-06-06). *Spray Polyurethane Foam (SPF) Insulation and How to Use it More Safely*. US EPA. Retrieved 2018-11-22.

Van Den Berg H, van der Ham L, Gutierrez H, Odu S, Roelofs T, and Weerdt JD (2012) Phosgene free route to Methyl Diphenyl Diisocyanate (MDI): A technical and economical evaluation. *Chem Eng J*; **207**: 254–257.

Viau C, Lafontaine M and Payan JP (2004) Creatinine normalization in biological monitoring revisited: the case of 1-hydroxypyrene. *Int Arch Occup Environ Health*; **77**: 177-185.

Vincentz Network GmbH & Co. KG. *Proposed restriction of diisocyanates*. European Coatings. Retrieved 2018-11-22.

Walker MJ (2007) Isocyanate Sampling and Analysis, *Ann Work Expo Health*; **51**: 645–646.

WATCH 2010, *WATCH Committee Biological Monitoring for isocyanates*. Available at http://www.hse.gov.uk/aboutus/hsc/iacs/acts/watch/051005/13.pdf. Accessed 19 December 2010.

Williams NR, Jones K and Cocker J (1999) Biological monitoring to assess exposure from isocyanate use in motor vehicle repair. *Occup Environ Med*; **56**: 598–601.

Wisnewski AV, Stowe MH, Nerlinger A, Opare-addo P, Decamp D, Kleinsmith CR, and Redlich CA (2012) Biomonitoring hexamethylene diisocyanate (HDI) exposure based on serum levels of HDI-specific IgG. *Ann Occup Hyg*; **56**: 901–910.

Wisnewski AV, Liu J, Redlich CA (2013) Connecting glutathione with immune responses to occupational methylene diphenyl diisocyanate exposure. *Chem. Biol. Interact*; **205**: 38–45.

Wisnewski AV, Nassar AF, Liu J, and Bello D (2019) Dilysine-Methylene Diphenyl Diisocyanate (MDI), a Urine Biomarker of MDI Exposure? *Chem Res Toxicol*; **32**: 557–565.

Wisnewski AV and Liu J (2022) Glutathione reactivity with aliphatic polyisocyanates. *PLoS ONE*; **17**: e0271471.

References

White J (2006a) Isocyanate exposure, emission and control in a small motor vehicle repair premises using spray rooms. White J, Coldwell M, Davies T, Helps J, Piney M Rimmer D, Saunders J and Wake D. HSE research report 496.

White J (2006b) *MDHS 25 Revisited; Development of MDHS 25/3, the Determination of Organic Isocyanates in Air.* Vol. 50, No. 1, pp. 15–27, 2006.

White J, Johnson P, Pengelly I, Keen C, and Coldwell M (2012) MDHS 25 Revisited Part 2, Modified Sampling and Analytical procedures Applied to HDI based Isocyanates. *Ann Occup Hyg*; **56**: 466–480.

Index

#

1-(2-methoxyphenyl), xvi, 49, 60, 67, 123, 125
1-(2-methoxyphenyl)-piperazine (1,2-MP), ix, xvi, 5, 6, 40, 41, 42, 49, 59, 60, 61, 62, 63, 65, 66, 67, 68, 70, 71
1-(2-methoxyphenyl)-piperazine (MOPIP), xvi, 5, 60
1-(2-pyridyl)-piperazine (1,2-PP), xvii, 59, 60
1-(9-anthracenylmethyl), xvi, 60, 67, 125
1-(9-anthracenylmethyl)piperazine (MAP), xvi, 59, 60, 67, 108, 125, 127
1,8-Diaminonaphtalene (DAN), xv, 67, 68, 71, 80, 119
3-(2-aminoethyl)indole, 67
8-hr-time weighted average, 19
9-(methylaminomethyl), 67

A

adhesives, v, vii, xi, 6, 9, 21, 57, 73, 78, 79, 80, 109, 110, 121
airborne monitoring, vi, 19, 57, 58, 80
American Conference of Governmental Industrial Hygienists (ACGIH), xv, 2, 19, 20, 21, 22, 73, 83, 84, 85, 87, 100, 119
American Industrial Hygiene Association (AIHA), xv, 48, 121
American Society for Testing and Materials (ASTM), xv, 129
analytical methods, vi, vii, xi, 29, 30, 40, 58, 59, 61, 63, 64, 66, 72, 80, 91, 96, 97, 100, 117, 120, 125, 132
Atmospheric Pressure Chemical Ionization (APCI), ix, xv, 29, 30, 39, 120
Australian Institute of Occupational Hygienists (AIOH), xiii, xv, 141
Australian National Occupational Safety and Health Commission (NOSHC), 20

B

biological exposure, xv, 21, 83, 85, 87, 119, 130
Biological Exposure Index (BEI), xv, 21, 87
Biological Guidance Value (BGV), xv
Biological Monitoring Guidance Value (BMGV), xv, 21, 24, 87
Biologische Arbeitsstoff Toleranzwerte (BAT) (biological tolerance values), xv, 21, 83, 103, 121, 122, 126
blood, 81, 89, 90, 100, 102, 116, 124

C

Certified Occupational Hygienist (COH), xv
Chemical Safety Reports (CSRs), xv, 73, 74, 75, 76, 77, 78
coatings, v, vii, xi, 6, 9, 73, 77, 79, 122, 133
common applications, v, 6, 53

D

Deutsche Forschungsgemeinschaft (DFG), xv, 21, 23, 83, 84, 85, 100, 121
Dibutylamine (DBA), xv, 5, 6, 42, 62, 64, 67, 68, 71
Diode Array Detector (DAD), xv, 40, 41, 42, 61

Index

E

Electrochemical Detection (ECD), vi, ix, xv, 29, 34, 35, 36, 40, 41, 49, 50, 51, 61, 62, 67, 96
Electrospray Ionisation (ESI), ix, xv, 29, 30, 39, 43, 47, 51, 120
engineering control(s), 15, 16, 17
Environmental Protection Agency, USA (EPA), xv, 22, 133
European Chemicals Agency (ECHA), xv, 22, 122
European Union (EU), xv, 15, 22, 26, 73, 81, 83, 84, 109, 122, 129
exposure, vi, vii, x, xi, xii, xiii, xvi, xvii, 2, 7, 8, 9, 11, 12, 13, 14, 15, 16, 17, 18, 19, 20, 21, 22, 23, 24, 25, 26, 27, 32, 39, 46, 48, 50, 57, 58, 59, 60, 64, 66, 67, 70, 71, 72, 73, 76, 77, 78, 79, 80, 81, 82, 83, 84, 85, 86, 87, 88, 89, 90, 91, 92, 98, 99, 100, 101, 102, 103, 104, 105, 106, 107, 108, 109, 110, 111, 112, 113, 114, 115, 116, 119, 120, 121, 122, 123, 124, 125, 126, 127, 128, 129, 130, 131, 132, 133, 134, 141
exposure control(s), v, xi, xii, 7, 12, 14, 16, 18, 21, 24, 26, 87, 125
exposure standards, v, xi, 19, 25, 85, 127

F

flame ionisation detection (FID), xv, 29, 32, 33, 34
fluorescence detection (FLD), xv, 60, 62, 63, 67
foam(s), ix, 1, 6, 7, 8, 17, 21, 68, 70, 71, 72, 73, 75, 76, 79, 89, 109, 110, 111, 112, 113, 119, 120, 121, 123, 125, 129, 130, 132, 133

G

gas chromatography (GC), vi, xv, 29, 32, 33, 34, 91, 119, 121, 123, 129, 130, 132, 133
gas chromatography (GC), ix, xv, 29, 30, 32, 33, 34, 36, 47, 51, 52, 53, 54, 94, 95, 96, 97, 100
German External QUality Assessment Scheme (G-EQUAS), xv, 49, 95, 96, 97

H

hazard statements, v, 12
Hazardous Chemical Information System (HCIS), xv, 132
Health & Safety Executive, UK (HSE), xvi, 6, 20, 21, 23, 35, 40, 49, 50, 51, 58, 59, 60, 61, 62, 63, 65, 66, 67, 69, 70, 72, 74, 75, 76, 77, 78, 80, 82, 84, 87, 100, 105, 122, 124, 127, 134
Health & Safety Laboratory, UK (HSL), xvi, 105, 124
Health Council of the Netherlands (HCOTN), xv, 123
health surveillance, v, ix, xi, 24, 25, 84, 86, 124, 126, 127
heterocumulene(s), 6
Hexamethylene Diamine (HDA), x, xv, 21, 47, 49, 87, 92, 93, 94, 95, 100, 101, 104, 105, 106, 107, 108, 123
Hexamethylene Diisocyanate (HDI), vii, x, xv, 1, 2, 6, 7, 9, 12, 20, 21, 43, 51, 57, 59, 60, 62, 66, 69, 72, 73, 74, 75, 77, 78, 79, 87, 91, 92, 96, 100, 101, 103, 104, 106, 108, 109, 116, 120, 121, 122, 123, 128, 129, 130, 133, 134
High-Performance Liquid Chromatography (HPLC), xvi, 34, 35, 36, 39, 40, 41, 51, 59, 60, 61, 62, 63, 67, 69, 71

I

industrial isocyanates, 7
inhalation exposure, 16, 17, 18, 26, 57, 72, 73, 74, 75, 76, 77, 78, 79, 80, 82, 86, 106, 116, 122, 126, 128
International Agency for Research on Cancer (IARC), xvi, 1, 23, 124

Index

International Electrotechnical Commission (IEC), xvi, 48, 120, 125
International Standards Organization (ISO), xvi, 23, 48, 58, 59, 60, 62, 63, 65, 66, 67, 68, 70, 80, 119, 120, 125, 128, 132
isocyanate(s), v, vi, xi, xiii, xvi, xvii, 1, 4, 6, 7, 8, 9, 11, 12, 13, 14, 15, 16, 17, 18, 19, 20, 21, 23, 25, 26, 29, 30, 32, 35, 36, 39, 40, 42, 46, 47, 49, 50, 51, 57, 58, 59, 60, 61, 62, 63, 64, 65, 66, 67, 69, 71, 72, 73, 74, 75, 78, 80, 81, 87, 88, 89, 90, 91, 92, 99, 100, 101, 103, 105, 108, 109, 113, 114, 116, 119, 120, 121, 123, 124, 125, 126, 128, 129, 130, 132, 133, 134
isocyanate functional group, vi, xvi, 1, 5, 19, 20, 26, 40, 42, 49, 51, 58, 59, 60, 61, 62, 63, 64, 66, 67, 68, 69, 70, 71, 72, 73, 75, 76, 77, 80, 108, 109, 112, 119, 128, 131, 132
Isophorone Diisocyanate (IPDI), xvi, 3, 7, 9, 12, 20, 21, 59, 91, 121

L

laboratory accreditation, vi, xi, 48, 49
Limit of Detection (LOD), xvi, 51, 62, 73, 96, 97, 106, 107, 112, 113
Limit of Quantitation (LOQ), xvi, 62, 69, 70, 73, 74, 75, 76, 77, 78, 79, 95, 96, 97, 104, 106, 107
liquid chromatography (LC), vi, ix, xvi, 29, 30, 31, 32, 34, 35, 36, 37, 38, 39, 40, 41, 42, 43, 44, 45, 46, 47, 50, 51, 52, 53, 54, 60, 63, 64, 67, 68, 69, 80, 91, 94, 95, 96, 97, 100, 102, 103, 119, 120, 123, 124, 125, 126, 127, 130, 131
Liquid Chromatography with Tandem Mass Spectrometry (LC-MS/MS), vi, ix, xvi, 36, 37, 38, 42, 43, 44, 45, 46, 47, 50, 54, 63, 64, 67, 68, 69, 80, 94, 95, 96, 97, 100, 102, 103
Liquid Chromatography–Mass Spectrometry (LC-MS), vi, ix, xvi, 29, 30, 31, 32, 36, 37, 38, 39, 42, 43, 44, 45, 46, 47, 50, 51, 52, 53, 54, 63, 64, 67, 68, 69, 80, 94, 95, 96, 97, 100, 102, 103, 130
Liquid-Liquid Extraction (LLE), xvi, 31, 93, 94
Litres per minute (L/min), xvi, 62

M

manufacturing, v, vii, xi, 7, 8, 73, 130
mass spectrometer (MS), vi, ix, xiii, xvi, 29, 30, 31, 32, 33, 34, 35, 36, 37, 38, 39, 40, 42, 43, 46, 47, 49, 50, 51, 52, 53, 54, 55, 62, 67, 69, 70, 71, 94, 95, 96, 97, 100, 120, 126, 127
Methods for the Determination of Hazardous Substance, HSE, UK (MDHS), xvi, 6, 35, 40, 49, 50, 51, 59, 60, 61, 62, 63, 65, 66, 67, 69, 70, 73, 80, 124, 127, 134
Methylene Diphenyl Diamine (MDA), xvi, 21, 47, 49, 86, 87, 89, 92, 93, 94, 95, 100, 103, 105, 110, 113, 114, 115, 125, 132
Methylene Diphenyl Isocyanate (MDI), vii, ix, x, xvi, 1, 4, 6, 7, 8, 9, 12, 19, 20, 21, 22, 23, 41, 43, 51, 57, 59, 60, 62, 65, 66, 68, 70, 71, 72, 73, 74, 75, 76, 77, 78, 79, 86, 87, 89, 91, 97, 100, 101, 102, 103, 104, 110, 113, 114, 115, 116, 119, 121, 123, 125, 126, 128, 129, 131, 133
micrograms (10^{-6} grams) per cubic metre ($\mu g/m^3$), xvii, 19, 20, 62, 74, 75, 79, 109
milligrams (10^{-3} grams) per cubic metre (mg/m^3), xvi
Motor Vehicle Repair (MVR), xvi, 16, 18, 104, 105, 106, 108, 109, 110
Multiple Reaction Monitoring (MRM), xvi, 37, 47, 51

Index

N

(N-methyl-aminomethyl)anthracene (MAMA), xvi, 62, 63, 67, 68
National Association of Testing Authorities, Australia (NATA), xvi, 141
National Institute for Occupational Safety and Health, USA (NIOSH), vi, xvi, 19, 20, 22, 23, 58, 59, 60, 61, 65, 66, 67, 72, 119, 127
National Institute of Standards and Technology, USA (NIST), xvi, 54
National Occupational Safety and Health Commission, Australia (NOHSC), xvi, 20, 85, 127
Nuclear Magnetic Resonance (NMR), xvi, 54

O

Occupational exposure limit(s) (OELs), x, xvi, 14, 19, 20, 82, 84, 85, 86, 88, 115, 124, 128
Occupational Safety & Health Agency, USA (OSHA), vi, xvi, 19, 20, 22, 23, 58, 59, 60, 61, 67, 68, 72, 83, 119, 128
oligomers, vi, vii, 1, 26, 27, 42, 57, 58, 59, 60, 62, 64, 65, 66, 68, 69, 71, 72, 78, 79, 80, 92, 101, 108, 109, 122, 128

P

parts per million (ppm), xvii, 19, 73
permissible exposure limits (PELs), xvi, 19, 22
personal protective equipment (PPE), xvii, 8, 13, 15, 16, 17, 18, 24, 82, 88, 115
Photodiode Array Detector (PDA), xvi, 35, 59, 94
p-nitrobenzyl-N-propylamine (Nitro reagent), xvi, 60, 67
Polytetrafluoroethylene (PTFE), xvii, 62, 63, 67

polyurethane (PU), v, vii, ix, xvii, 6, 7, 8, 9, 13, 17, 21, 57, 65, 68, 70, 71, 72, 73, 74, 75, 78, 79, 119, 120, 121, 123, 125, 126, 129, 130, 132, 133
production, v, xi, 2, 5, 6, 7, 8, 73, 74, 75, 89, 109, 110, 111, 113, 114, 119, 122, 125
Proficiency Analytical Testing (PAT), xvi, 49
proficiency test (PT), xvii, 30, 48, 49, 116
PU adhesives, 9, 78

Q

Quality Assurance (QA), xvii
Quality Control (QC), vi, xvii, 48
Quality Control/Quality Assurance (QC/QA), xvii

R

reactivity, v, xi, 5, 30, 67, 102, 103, 133
respiratory protective equipment (RPE), 17, 18, 19, 23, 89, 111, 114

S

Safe Work Australia (SWA), xvii, 12, 85, 130, 132
safety data sheet (SDS), xvii, 11, 14, 82, 121, 122
sampling, vi, vii, ix, xi, 5, 6, 12, 23, 24, 29, 30, 40, 57, 58, 59, 60, 62, 63, 64, 65, 66, 67, 68, 69, 70, 71, 72, 80, 82, 84, 88, 90, 98, 99, 104, 105, 108, 119, 122, 123, 125, 126, 127, 128, 129, 132, 133, 134
Scientific Committee on Occupational Exposure Limits (SCOEL), xvii, 84, 85, 122
short-term exposure limit (STEL), xvii, 2, 20
Solid Phase Extraction (SPE), xvii, 31, 93, 94, 96, 97
spray foam, v, vii, 8, 65, 66, 70, 71, 73, 76, 79, 115, 126, 128

Index

T

Threshold Limit Value (TLV), xvii, 2, 19, 20, 22, 73, 84, 119
Time Weighted Average (TEA), xvii
Time-of-Flight (TOF), xvii, 39
Toluene Diamine (TDA), xvii, 21, 47, 49, 92, 93, 94, 95, 100, 105, 110, 111, 112, 123, 125
Toluene Diisocyanate (TDI), vii, ix, xvii, 1, 3, 6, 7, 8, 9, 12, 19, 20, 21, 22, 23, 41, 43, 57, 59, 60, 68, 71, 72, 73, 74, 75, 77, 78, 79, 80, 87, 91, 95, 96, 100, 101, 109, 110, 111, 112, 119, 123, 124, 125, 126, 129
Total Reactive Isocyanate Group (TRIG), xvii, 19, 67, 80, 119

U

ultra-performance liquid chromatography, xvii
ultra-violet (UV), vi, ix, xvii, 34, 35, 36, 37, 40, 41, 42, 49, 50, 59, 60, 61, 63, 67, 69, 71

United Kingdom (UK), xiii, xvi, xvii, 19, 20, 21, 58, 59, 61, 62, 63, 68, 73, 75, 76, 77, 82, 83, 84, 104, 106, 107, 110, 111, 112, 113, 119, 121, 124, 125, 127, 129
United Kingdom (UK) (UPLC), xvii, 20, 82
United Kingdom Health and Safety Executive (UK-HSE), 20
United States of America (USA), xv, xvi, xvii, 19, 20, 22, 58, 59, 60, 81, 104, 106, 119, 127, 128, 133

V

vapour pressure, 1, 57, 75
vapour(s), 1, 13, 14, 15, 16, 23, 57, 58, 61, 62, 63, 64, 65, 66, 70, 71, 75, 129

W

Workplace Exposure Standard (WES), xvii, 82, 85, 130, 132

About the Author

Jimmy Hu, PhD is a senior occupational & analytical chemist at SafeWork NSW in the area of occupational and chemical exposure analysis. He received a PhD from the University of Newcastle and has since worked at Lehigh University in Pennsylvania and Monash University in Victoria as a post-doc in the early 2000's. Since 2004, Jimmy has worked at SafeWork NSW on a range of projects focusing on work exposures and health. His interests include developing and using sophisticated techniques to analyse biological samples for trace levels of toxic substances and their metabolites. Further, he also has over 20 years' of experience in the field of workplace air monitoring. His work on biological and air monitoring to assess exposure to isocyanates in motor vehicle repair was recognised internationally and he is considered one of the leading experts in the field in Australia.

Jimmy Hu has published one book chapter and over 50 scientific papers and technical reports, including in the *Annals of Work Exposures and Health* and *Journal of Analytical Toxicology*. Jimmy is an editorial board member of the *Journal of Health Safety and Environment*, a member of Standards Australia Committee EV-007 "Methods for Examination of Air", a technical assessor of the National Association of Testing Authorities (NATA), and a full member of the Australian Institute of Occupational Hygienists (AIOH).

Email: jimmy.hu@safework.nsw.gov.au